Surgical Critical Care

For the MRCS OSCE

Second Edition

Mazyar Kanani PhD FRCS
Consultant Cardiothoracic Surgeon, Cardiac Unit,
Great Ormond Street Hospital, London, UK

Simon Lammy MRCS(Ed) PgDip(Oxon)
ST2 Neurological Surgery (Neurosurgery),
Institute of Neurological Sciences,
Southern General Hospital,
Glasgow, UK

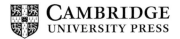

CAMBRIDGE
UNIVERSITY PRESS

CAMBRIDGE
UNIVERSITY PRESS

University Printing House, Cambridge CB2 8BS, United Kingdom

Cambridge University Press is part of the University of Cambridge.

It furthers the University's mission by disseminating knowledge in the pursuit of education, learning and research at the highest international levels of excellence.

www.cambridge.org
Information on this title: www.cambridge.org/9781107657687

First published 2003 by Greenwich Medical Media
Reprinted 2004
Reprinted 2005 by Cambridge University Press
Second edition 2015

Printed in the United Kingdom by TJ International Ltd. Padstow Cornwall

A catalogue record for this publication is available from the British Library

Library of Congress Cataloguing in Publication data
Kanani, Mazyar, author.
[Surgical critical care vivas]
Surgical critical care for the MRCS OSCE / Mazyar Kanani, Simon Lammy. – Second edition.
  p. ; cm.
Preceded by: Surgical critical care vivas / Mazyar Kanani. 2003.
Includes bibliographical references and index.
ISBN 978-1-107-65768-7 (paperback : alk.)
I. Lammy, Simon, author.   II. Title.
[DNLM: 1. Critical Care–Examination Questions.   2. Surgical Procedures,
Operative–Examination Questions.   WO 18.2]
RC86.9
616.02′8076 – dc23   2015012526

ISBN 978-1-107-65768-7 Paperback

Cambridge University Press has no responsibility for the persistence or accuracy
of URLs for external or third-party internet websites referred to in this publication,
and does not guarantee that any content on such websites is, or will remain,
accurate or appropriate.

. . . .

Dedicated to Florence Michaela Eibhlin Kanani

Mazyar Kanani

Dedicated to my mum, Joanne, my father, Victor,
and my brother, James

Simon Lammy

CONTENTS

ACKNOWLEDGEMENTS

This project would not have been possible without the support of Joanna Chamberlin and Ross Higman, editorial staff at Cambridge University Press, whose enthusiasm for a second edition proved highly encouraging. Simon Lammy also wishes to express his gratitude to Mazyar Kanani for permitting him to revise and reorganise the book, following his proposal in June 2012 as an FY2 in Aberdeen, having previously used the first edition to successfully pass the MRCS Part B OSCE.

ABBREVIATIONS

AAA	Abdominal aortic aneurysm
ABCDE	Airway, breathing, circulation, disability, exposure
ABG	Arterial blood gas
ABPA	Allergic bronchopulmonary aspergillosis
ACA	Anterior cerebral artery
ACTH	Adrenocorticotropic hormone
ADH	Antidiuretic hormone
ADP	Adenosine diphosphate
AF	Atrial fibrillation
AIDS	Acquired immunodeficiency syndrome
AKI	Acute kidney injury
ALI	Acute lung injury
ALS	Advanced Life Support
AMP	Adenosine monophosphate
APTT	Activated partial thromboplastin time
$APTT_r$	Activated partial thromboplastin time ratio
ARDS	Acute respiratory distress syndrome
ASA	American Society of Anesthesiologists
ATD	Adult therapeutic dose
ATLS®	Advanced Trauma Life Support®
ATN	Acute tubular necrosis

ATP	Adenosine triphosphate
AV	Atrioventricular/arteriovenous
AVRT	Atrioventricular re-entry tachycardia
BAL	Bronchoalveolar lavage
BBB	Blood–brain barrier
BM	Boehringer Mannheim
BMI	Body mass index
BP	Blood pressure
2,3-BPG	2,3-bisphosphoglycerate
BSA	Body surface area
BTS	British Thoracic Society
CCrISP®	Care of the Critically Ill Surgical Patient
CCU	Coronary care unit
cGMP	Cyclic guanosine monophosphate
CI	Cardiac index
CK	Creatinine kinase
CKD	Chronic kidney disease
CMV	Cytomegalovirus
CO	Cardiac output/carbon monoxide
CO_2	Carbon dioxide
COAD	Chronic obstructive airways disease
COPD	Chronic obstructive pulmonary disease
COX	Cyclooxygenase
CPAP	Continuous positive airways pressure
CPP	Cerebral perfusion pressure
CPR	Cardiopulmonary resuscitation
CRT	Capillary refill time
CSF	Cerebrospinal fluid
CT	Computed tomography

CTPA	CT pulmonary angiography
CUS	Compression ultrasonography
CVC	Central venous catheter
CVP	Central venous pressure
CXR	Chest radiograph
dAg	Direct antiglobulin test
DBD	Donation after brainstem death
DCD	Donation after circulatory death
DHTR	Delayed haemolytic transfusion reaction
DI	Diabetes insipidus
DIC	Disseminated intravascular coagulation
DKA	Diabetic ketoacidosis
*DL*co	Transfer factor
DP	Diastolic pressure
DPL	Diagnostic peritoneal lavage
DSA	Digital subtraction angiography
DVT	Deep venous thrombosis
ECF	Extracellular fluid
ECG	Electrocardiogram/graph
ECMO	Extracorporeal membrane oxygenation
EDH	Extradural haematoma
EDRF	Endothelium-derived relaxing factor
EEG	Electroencephalogram/graph
EF	Ejection fraction
eGFR	Estimated glomerular filtration rate
ELISA	Enzyme-linked immunosorbent assay
ERV	Expiratory reserve volume
ESR	Erythrocyte sedimentation rate
ESRF	End-stage renal failure

EVD	External ventricular drain
EWS	Early Warning Score
FAST	Focused assessment with sonography in trauma
FBC	Full blood count
FEV_1	Forced expiratory volume in 1 second
FFA	Free fatty acids
FFP	Fresh frozen plasma
FiO_2	Fraction of inspired oxygen
FNHTR	Febrile non-haemolytic transfusion reaction
FRC	Functional residual capacity
FVC	Forced vital capacity
GBS	Guillan-Barré syndrome
GCS	Glasgow Coma Scale
GFR	Glomerular filtration rate
GI	Gastrointestinal
GMC	General Medical Council
HAS	Human albumin solution
Hb	Haemoglobin
HBsAg	Hepatitis B surface antigen
HBV	Hepatitis B virus
Hct	Haematocrit
HCV	Hepatitis C virus
HDU	High dependency unit
HITS	Heparin-induced thrombocytopaenia syndrome
HIV	Human immunodeficiency virus
HLA	Human leucocyte antigen
HPA	Human platelet antigen
HR	Heart rate

HRT	Hormone replacement therapy
5-HT	5-hydroxy-tryptamine
HTLV	Human T-cell lymphocyte virus
IABP	Intra-arterial blood pressure/intra-arterial balloon pump counter-pulsation
IC	Inspiratory capacity
ICP	Intracranial pressure
ICU	Intensive care unit
I:E	Inspiratory:expiratory ratio
Ig	Immunoglobulin
IHD	Ischaemic heart disease
IIH	Idiopathic intracranial hypertension
IL	Interleukin
IM	Intramuscular
IMV	Intermittent mandatory ventilation
IN	Intranasal
INH	Inhalation
INR	International normalised ratio
IO	Intraosseus
IPPV	Intermittent positive pressure ventilation
IRV	Inspiratory reserve volume
IT	Intrathecal
IV	Intravenous
JVP	Jugular venous pulse/pressure
Kco	Transfer coefficient
LA	Local anaesthetic
LBBB	Left bundle branch block
LDH	Lactate dehydrogenase
LFTs	Liver function tests

LMWH	Low molecular weight heparin
LP	Lumbar puncture
LVEDV	Left ventricular end-diastolic volume
MAHA	Microangiopathic haemolytic anaemia
MAP	Mean arterial pressure
MI	Myocardial infarction
MND	Motor neurone disease
MODS	Multi-organ dysfunction syndrome
MPAP	Mean pulmonary artery pressure
MRI	Magnetic resonance imaging
MRSA	Methicillin-resistant *Staphylococcus aureus*
NAIT	Neonatal alloimmune thrombocytopaenia
NAT	Nucleic acid testing
NG	Nasogastric
NIBP	Non-invasive blood pressure
NJ	Nasojejunal
NO	Nitric oxide
NSAIDs	Non-steroidal anti-inflammatory drugs
O_2	Oxygen
OCP	Oral contraceptive pill
PA	Pulmonary artery
$PaCO_2$	Partial arterial pressure of carbon dioxide
PACWP	Pulmonary artery capillary wedge pressure
PAF	Platelet-activating factor
PAFC	Pulmonary artery flotation catheter
PaO_2	Arterial partial pressure of oxygen
PAS	Platelet additive solution
PCA	Patient-controlled analgesia/posterior cerebral artery

PCC	Prothrombin complex concentrate
PCI	Percutaneous coronary intervention
pCO_2	Partial pressure of carbon dioxide
PDE	Phosphodiesterase
PE	Pulmonary thromboembolism
PEA	Pulseless electrical activity
PEEP	Positive end-expiratory pressure
PEFR	Peak expiratory flow rate
PEG	Percutaneous endoscopic gastrostomy
PET	Positron emission tomography
PFO	Patent foramen ovale
PFTs	Pulmonary function tests
PG	Prostaglandin
PICC	Peripherally inserted central catheter
pO_2	Partial pressure of oxygen
PP	Pulse pressure
PPIs	Proton pump inhibitors
PSV	Pressure support ventilation
PT	Prothrombin time
PTH	Parathyroid hormone
PTHrP	Parathyroid hormone-related peptide
PTP	Post-transfusion purpuric reaction
PVR	Pulmonary vascular resistance
RAA	Renin–angiotensin–aldosterone
rAAA	Ruptured abdominal aortic aneurysm
Rh	Rhesus
RIG	Radiologically inserted gastrostomy
RV	Residual volume
SA	Sinoatrial

SAG-M	Saline, adenine, glucose and mannitol
SAH	Subarachnoid haemorrhage
SaO_2	Arterial oxygen saturation
SC	Subcutaneous
SD-FFP	Solvent detergent fresh frozen plasma
SDH	Subdural haematoma
SEWS	Scottish Early Warning Score
SIADH	Syndrome of inappropriate ADH secretion
SIMV	Synchronised intermittent mandatory ventilation
SIRS	Systemic inflammatory response syndrome
SLE	Systemic lupus erythematosus
SP	Systolic pressure
SPECT	Single photon emission computed tomography
STEMI	ST-segment elevated myocardial infarction
SV	Stroke volume
SVC	Superior vena cava
SvO_2	Mixed venous oxygen saturation
SVR	Systemic vascular resistance
SVT	Supraventricular tachycardia
$T°$	Temperature
TACO	Transfusion-associated circulatory overload
TA-GvHD	Transfusion-associated graft vs. host disease
TB	Tuberculosis
TC	Transcutaneous
TCD	Transcranial Doppler
TEDS	Thromboembolic deterrent stockings
TEE	Transoesophageal echocardiography
TGF-β	Transforming growth factor beta

TLC	Total lung capacity
TLV	Total lung volume
TNF	Tumour necrosis factor
TOE	Transoesophageal echocardiography
TPN	Total parenteral nutrition
TRALI	Transfusion-related acute lung injury
TT	Thrombin time
TTE	Transthoracic echocardiography
TURP	Transurethral resection of the prostate
TV	Tidal volume
U&Es	Urea & electrolytes
US	Ultrasound
VA	Alveolar ventilation
VAD	Ventricular-assist device
VAP	Ventilator-associated pneumonia
VATS	Video-assisted thoracoscopic surgery
VC	Vital capacity
vCJD	Variant Creutzfeldt–Jakob disease
VKA	Vitamin K antagonist
VP	Ventriculoperitoneal
V/Q	Ventilation/perfusion ratio
VSD	Ventricular septal defect
VT	Ventricular tachycardia
vWF	von Willebrand's factor
WHO	World Health Organisation
WPW	Wolff–Parkinson–White

Ward care (level 0–2)

Chapter 1

Airway

Assessment

Airway assessment

How is the airway assessed clinically?

Assessment is based on the principle of: Look, Listen and Feel.

- *Look*: for the presence of accessory muscles of respiration (neck, shoulders, chest and abdomen) being used, presence of obvious foreign bodies in the airway, facial/airway injury and the 'see-saw' pattern of complete airway obstruction (NB. central cyanosis is a late sign)
- *Listen*: for the presence of inspiratory stridor, as this indicates upper airways obstruction (laryngeal level and above). Also take note of grunting, gurgling (liquid or semi-solid foreign matter in the upper airways) and snoring sounds (indicating the pharynx is partially occluded by the tongue or palate). Expiratory wheeze suggests lower airways obstruction. Crowing indicates laryngeal spasm
- *Feel*: for chest wall movements and airflow at the nose and mouth (for 10 seconds)

Note that in cases of trauma, the assessment has to be performed with cervical spine (C-spine) control.

What techniques of airway management do you know?

Broadly speaking there are *simple* and *definitive* airway management techniques that increase in complexity if previous measures fail

- Simple measures
    - *Basic airway manoeuvres*: these include a head tilt, chin lift and jaw thrust, which open up the airway and permit the use of rigid suction devices (Yankauer sucker) to clear secretions and forceps (Magill) to remove solid debris
    - *Basic airway adjuncts*: these include nasopharyngeal and oropharyngeal airways. If a patient tolerates an oropharyngeal, then it is prudent to request an anaesthetic review as the airway is at risk of imminent collapse
- Complex measures
    - *Endotracheal intubation*: this requires anaesthetic expertise and can be achieved through the mouth (orotracheal) or the nose (nasotracheal) intubation
    - *Surgical airway*: this requires a cut down through tissues in the neck and can be achieved in three ways (*see* Airway Adjuncts)

How are the head tilt, chin lift and jaw thrust manoeuvres performed?

- *Head tilt*: the hand is placed on the patient's forehead and another under the occipital protuberance to tilt the head back gently
- *Chin lift*: the fingers of one hand are placed under the mandible in the mid-line and then lifted upwards to bring the chin forward

- *Jaw thrust*: the angles of the mandible are identified on both sides, the index and middle fingers are placed behind it and a steady upwards and forwards pulling pressure is applied to lift the mandible (this is painful, and if a patient tolerates it, consider an anaesthetic review). Finally, the thumbs are used to slightly open the mouth by downward displacement of the chin

These simple positional methods are successful in most cases where airway obstruction is caused by loss of muscle tone in the pharynx. Always check for success after each manoeuvre using the Look, Listen and Feel sequence.

Basic concepts

Oxygen: basic physiology

What is the FiO_2 of atmospheric air?
0.21. Since 21% of the atmosphere is made up of oxygen.

What is meant by the oxygen cascade?
This describes the incremental and successive drops in the pO_2 from the atmosphere to the arterial circulation.

What are the changes in the oxygen cascade?
- *Atmospheric air*: $pO_2 = 21.0$ kPa
- *Tracheal air*: $pO_2 = 19.8$ kPa
- *Alveolar gas*: $pO_2 = 14.0$ kPa
- *Arterial blood gas*: $pO_2 = 13.3$ kPa

How is oxygen transported in the body?

Oxygen is transported by binding to haemoglobin (99%) or dissolved in solution (1%).

What does Henry's law state, and how is this used to calculate the amount of oxygen dissolved in the blood?

Henry's law states that the *gas content* of a *solution* is equal to the *product* of the *solubility* and the *partial pressure* of the *gas*. At 37°C the solubility of oxygen in blood is 0.03 ml/L for every mmHg rise in the partial pressure ($0.03 \times PaO_2$).

What is haemoglobin composed of?

Haemoglobin is a globular protein consisting of a haem component and a globin chain. The haem moiety consists of Fe^{2+} and a protoporphyrin ring. The globin chain consists of two α- and two β-chains together and a 2,3-bisphosphoglycerate (2,3-BPG) molecule in an adult. A total of four oxygen molecules are able to bind to each globin molecule.

What other molecules may bind to haemoglobin under normal circumstances?

- *Carbon dioxide*: this binds to the globin chain forming a carbamino compound
- *Protons (H^+)*: these specifically bind to amino, carboxyl and imidazole groups in the globin chain
- *2,3-BPG*: this is a by-product of red cell metabolism. It is able to form covalent bonds with the β-subunits, wedging them apart in the de-oxygenated state

Where are the main sites of haemopoesis?
- *Yolk sac*: in the first few weeks of gestation
- *Bone marrow*: from the first few weeks after birth
- *Liver and spleen*: most important sites up until the first 7 months of gestation. The adult can revert to these sites in pathological states – so-called 'extramedullary haemopoesis'

What is the life span of a red blood cell?
The average life span is 120 days, after which it is broken down in the reticuloendothelial system.

Draw the oxygen dissociation curve and label the axis

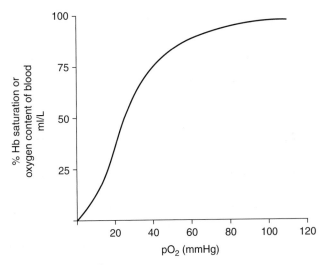

Figure 1.1

What accounts for the shape of the curve?

The sigmoidal curve reflects the progressive nature with which each oxygen molecule binds to haemoglobin. This binding is termed *cooperative* – the binding of one oxygen molecule facilitates the bind of the next.

What is the Bohr Effect and what causes it?

The Bohr Effect is a *shift* of the dissociation curve to the *right*, signifying a reduction of the oxygen affinity of the molecule and, therefore, a greater tendency to off-load oxygen into the tissues. This *right shift* can be caused by

- Increased temperature
- Increased acidity
- Increased 2,3-BPG (e.g. due to chronic hypoxia)
- Hypercarbia

What physiological effect does it have?

It ensures greater and more ready tissue oxygenation during states of acute or chronic reduction in tissue perfusion.

How does the oxygen dissociation curve in the foetus compare to that of the adult and what accounts for this difference?

The foetal oxygen dissociation curve is shifted to the *left*. This reflects the increased oxygen affinity of foetal haemoglobin caused by the presence of the γ-subunit (instead of the β) that cannot form covalent bonds with 2,3-BPG. This ensures that it is readily able to take up oxygen from the maternal haemoglobin molecule.

How much oxygen is bound to haemoglobin when fully saturated?

When fully saturated each gram of haemoglobin can bind to 1.34 ml of oxygen. It follows that the oxygen-carrying capacity of the blood is $1.34 \times$ [Hb] at full (100%) saturation.

Therefore on what factors does the total amount of oxygen in the blood depend? How is this calculated?

O_2 content of blood

$=$ amount bound to Hb + amount dissolved in blood

or

$= (1.34 \times [Hb] \times \text{% saturation}) + (0.03 \times PaO_2)$

The factors determining the total oxygen content of the blood are

- [Hb]
- (%) saturation of the molecule
- PaO_2
- T°, as this determines the oxygen solubility (although in practice this is of little significance)

The total is in the order of 200 ml/L for arterial blood at 97% saturation.

Carbon dioxide: basic physiology

What is the $FiCO_2$ of atmospheric air?

0.00035. Since 0.035% of the atmosphere is made up of carbon dioxide.

What are the changes in the carbon dioxide cascade?

- *Atmospheric air*: $pCO_2 = 0.03$ kPa
- *Alveolar air*: $pCO_2 = 5.30$ kPa
- *Arterial blood gas*: $pCO_2 = 5.30$ kPa
- *Venous blood gas*: $pCO_2 = 6.10$ kPa
- *Exhaled air*: $pCO_2 = 4.00$ kPa

Why is there virtually no alveolar–arterial pCO_2 difference, unlike oxygen?

Carbon dioxide has a very high water solubility compared to oxygen and rapidly diffuses across the respiratory epithelium.

Under what conditions does this difference increase?

Under the pathological conditions of a ventilation/perfusion mismatch and when there is an increase in CO_2 production.

How is carbon dioxide transported in the body?

- *Bicarbonate ions (HCO_3^-)*: accounts for 85–90% of carriage
- *Carbamino compounds*: formed when CO_2 binds with the terminal amino group of plasma proteins. Five-to-ten per cent of CO_2 is transported in this way
- *Physically dissolved in solution*: this accounts for 5%

How does the mode of CO_2 transport differ between arterial and venous blood?

In arterial blood there is *less* carbamino compound carriage and *more* bicarbonate carriage. The amount physically dissolved varies little between the two circulations. This variation is due to the difference in pH affecting the binding and dissociation properties of the molecule.

How does the amount of CO_2 physically dissolved in plasma compare to the amount of dissolved oxygen?

Only $\sim$1% of oxygen in blood is dissolved in plasma. This value is much lower than CO_2 ($\sim$5%) because oxygen is 24 times less water soluble.

You mentioned that CO_2 combines with plasma proteins to form carbamino compounds. What is the most significant of these plasma proteins?

Haemoglobin, as CO_2 binds to its globin chain.

How does CO_2 come to be carried as the bicarbonate ion?

$$CO_2 + H_2O = H_2CO_3 = H^+ + HCO_3^-$$

This interchangeable reaction is catalysed by the enzyme *carbonic anhydrase.*

What happens to all of the H^+ generated by this process?

This is 'mopped up' by other buffer systems. The H^+ binds with the haemoglobin molecule, mainly the imidazole groups of the polypeptide chain, and is therefore buffered.

What effect does this buffering have on the transport of oxygen by haemoglobin?

The addition of the H^+ and CO_2 to the haemoglobin chain leads to a reduced oxygen affinity. This is seen as a *right* shift in the oxygen dissociation curve.

What happens to the bicarbonate generated in the red cell when it carries CO_2?

It diffuses out of the red cell and into the plasma (unlike H^+ it is able to penetrate the red cell membrane). The electrochemical neutrality is maintained by a Cl^- ion entering as an HCO_3^- leaves, and this is known as the *chloride shift*.

How does the transport of CO_2 affect the osmotic balance of a red cell?

The bicarbonate and chloride generated following CO_2 carriage by the red cell increases the intracellular osmotic pressure. This causes the cell to swell as extra H_2O diffuses through the cell membrane, which is why the haematocrit (Hct) of venous blood is 3% higher than arterial blood.

How does the shape of the O_2 dissociation curve differ from the CO_2 dissociation curve?

- The CO_2 dissociation curve is *curvilinear*
- The O_2 dissociation curve is *sigmoidal*

Why cannot the amount of CO_2 in the blood be expressed as a *percentage-saturation*, unlike the case for oxygen?

This is because CO_2 is more water soluble than oxygen and never reaches a saturation point. Its blood saturation cannot reasonably be expressed as a percentage of a total level. This can be seen in the CO_2 dissociation curve – it never reaches a peak, but continues to rise in linear fashion.

What is the difference between the Bohr Effect and the Haldane Effect?

- The Bohr Effect describes the changes in the affinity of the haemoglobin chain for oxygen following variations in the $PaCO_2$, H^+ and $T°$
- The Haldane Effect describes changes in the affinity of the blood for CO_2 as the PaO_2 changes. As the PaO_2 *increases* the affinity of the blood for CO_2 *decreases*. This is seen as a *downward* shift in the CO_2 dissociation curve

Which equation defines the relationship between PaO_2 and $PaCO_2$?

The relationship is given by the *alveolar gas equation* (in simplified form)

$$PaO_2 = PiO_2 - PaCO_2/R$$

This translates as $PiO_2 =$ inspired pO_2 and $R =$ respiratory exchange ratio, which is normally 0.8.

Oxygen: therapy

How may oxygen be delivered to the patient?

- *Variable performance devices*: the FiO_2 delivered depends on the flow rate
  - *Nasal cannulae*: a convenient way for the patient

- *Face mask (Hudson mask)*: at 2 L/min the FiO_2 achieved is 0.25–0.30. At 6–10 L/min the FiO_2 equals 0.30–0.40

If the flow is not high enough, then re-breathing of air exhaled into the mask occurs, leading to hypercarbia.

- *Fixed performance devices*: there is a constant FiO_2 delivered so the desired amount can be administered accurately
  - *Venturi mask*: oxygen flows through a device that entrains air from the side holes at a certain rate. The degree of air mixing within the device produces the desired FiO_2
  - *Reservoir bag (non-re-breath mask)*: this is attached onto the end of a face mask. During tachypnoea the patient inhales directly from the oxygen in the bag so that the FiO_2 is close to 1.0. This is used in the trauma setting to deliver as much oxygen as possible
  - *Continuous positive pressure ventilation*: this ensures that the small airways do not collapse at the end of expiration by providing a positive pressure through the respiratory cycle
  - *Invasive respiratory support*: this requires intubation to enable intermittent positive pressure ventilation

What is the danger of oxygen therapy in the chronic CO_2-retaining patient and what is the pathophysiology?
In patients who chronically retain CO_2, uncontrolled use of oxygen, may induce apnoea. There are two main explanations

- *Loss of hypoxic pulmonary drive*: those who have a chronically raised CO_2 rely on hypoxia to stimulate respiration. If this is abolished by the use of oxygen, then apnoea may be the result. To decrease this, in a non-trauma situation, the patient should initially be given 24% oxygen through a Venturi mask, which is steadily increased depending on the effect

- *Abolition of hypoxia*: this can reverse the normal compensatory hypoxic pulmonary vasoconstriction. This leads to a deteriorating V/Q mismatch

What are the other potential problems associated with oxygen therapy?

- *Absorption atelectasis*: in the absence of nitrogen (which by its slow absorption 'splints' the airways open), oxygen is absorbed rapidly from the alveolus, causing the airways to collapse after it
- *Pulmonary toxicity*: oxygen irritates the mucosa of the airways directly leading to loss of surfactant and progressive fibrosis
- *Risk of fires and explosions*: oxygen supports combustion

Oxygen: monitoring (pulse oximetry)

What is pulse oximetry and what does it measure?

Pulse oximetry is a non-invasive and continuous method of assessing arterial oxygen saturation (SaO_2) and pulse rate. The fingertip and ear lobe are common sites that are used. It is not a measure of the total oxygen content of the blood or the PaO_2. It does not assess ventilation, which requires a measure of the $PaCO_2$.

By which principle does pulse oximetry work?

Pulse oximetry works on the principles of spectrophotometry. It contains a probe emitting light (LED) at the red (660 nm) and infra-red (940 nm) wavelengths and a photodetector (photodiode).

It relies on the differing amount of light absorbed by the saturated and unsaturated Hb molecules. The percentage oxygen saturation of the blood is calculated from the ratio of these two forms of the molecule.

What are its disadvantages and sources of error?

Problems encountered include

- Diminished accuracy below a saturation of ~70%
- There is a delay of ~20 seconds between actual and displayed values (though more modern probes might have much shorter delays). This limits its use in the emergency setting
- Poor peripheral perfusion (e.g. during haemorrhagic shock) and ambient light pollution leads to a poor signal quality
- Abnormal pigments affect the results. Extrinsic pigments include nail varnish. Intrinsic pigments include bilirubin of the jaundiced patient, methaemoglobin and carboxyhaemoglobin. Jaundice underestimates the true SaO_2 and carbon monoxide poisoning overestimates the true SaO_2. There is no interference from polycythaemia or foetal haemoglobin
- Abnormal pulsations such as cardiac arrhythmia or venous pulsations of right heart valve defects may interfere with the signal, so be sceptical and consider arterial blood gas (ABG) analysis

What is methaemoglobin?

This is a haemoglobin molecule that contains iron in the ferric (Fe^{3+}) state within its haem portion, as opposed to the normal ferrous (Fe^{2+}) state. It may be due to a congenital deficiency of reducing enzymes, or acquired through exposure to various chemicals such as the local anaesthetic agent prilocaine.

The molecule is less able to carry oxygen and patients may appear cyanotic owing to the darker colour of methaemoglobin. It may be treated with the use of a reducing agent such as methylene blue.

How may ventilation be assessed?

Ventilation, which is a measure of the ability to 'blow off' CO_2 adequately, may be measured and displayed visually by capnography. The end-tidal CO_2 is detected by a sensor placed at the exhaled stream of air. Owing to the relatively high solubility of CO_2, this is a good measure of the $PaCO_2$ when the ventilation and perfusion are well matched.

Capnography may also be used to assess airway patency and in the detection of oesophageal intubation.

Procedures

Airway adjuncts

What do you know of the airway adjuncts?

These simple airway adjuncts are often essential to maintain an open airway, and the position of the head and neck should be maintained (*see* basic airway manoeuvres) to keep the airway aligned. The nasopharyngeal and oropharyngeal airways are designed to overcome soft palate obstruction and backward tongue displacement.

- *Nasopharyngeal airway*: this is a tube bevelled at one end, having a stopper fashioned at the other end (no need for a safety pin)
  - It is tolerated in conscious patients
  - Insertion used to be completely contraindicated in skull base (or cribriform plate) fractures due to inadvertent insertion through a fracture into the cranial vault, but this is an extremely rare occurrence. If a skull base fracture is suspected, an oropharyngeal airway is preferred, but if this is not possible, and the airway is obstructed, gentle insertion of a nasopharyngeal airway may be life-saving
  - It comes in sizes 6–7 mm, which are suitable for adults
  - Insertion can cause damage to nasal mucosa, resulting in bleeding, and if the tube is too long, it may stimulate the laryngeal or glossopharyngeal reflexes to cause laryngospasm and vomiting
- *Oropharyngeal airway*: this is a curved plastic tube, flanged and reinforced at the oral end, and the stopper is flattened so the teeth can bite into it
  - It is not tolerated in conscious patients
  - Insertion is contraindicated if a gag reflex is present and use of a nasopharyngeal airway is preferable. If it is tolerated, this indicates a significant decrease in GCS and imminent airway compromise (so request an anaesthetic review to secure the airway)
  - It comes in sizes 2, 3 and 4 (small, medium and large), which are suitable for most adults

- Insertion can occasionally push the tongue backwards, exacerbating obstruction, and it may also lodge in the vallecula or the epiglottis. Laryngospasm and vomiting may occur if inserted in a conscious patient, if glossopharyngeal and laryngeal reflexes are present

How are the nasopharyngeal and oropharyngeal airways inserted?

- *Nasopharyngeal airway*: check for right nostril patency, attach safety pin to end of tube (if needed) and lubricate the tip, insert it bevel end first and perpendicular to orifice (towards the ear). Once in place, reassess the airway according to Look, Listen and Feel
- *Oropharyngeal airway*: open the mouth employing basic airway manoeuvres. Suction out debris and insert it upside down (curved side pointing to the palate). Rotate it 180° between the hard and soft palate and seat the flattened section between the gums and teeth

What kinds of surgical airway are there?

There are three types of surgical airway

- Needle cricothyroidotomy (and jet insufflations of oxygen)
- Cricothyroidotomy
- Tracheostomy, which may be performed in the emergency or elective setting

What are the indications for a surgical airway?

- Failed intubation, e.g. due to oedema
- Traumatic fracture of the larynx

In which anatomic location are the surgical airways sited?

Both types of cricothyroidotomy are performed through the median cricothyroid ligament. This is the thickened anterior portion of the cricothyroid membrane that runs between the cricoid and thyroid cartilages. A tracheostomy may be placed from the 2nd to 5th tracheal rings (*see* Chapter 6, Tracheostomy).

How is jet insufflation of oxygen performed, and what is the main precaution to be considered?

This is carried out by way of a needle passed into the airway through the median cricothyroid ligament. It is connected to a source of oxygen via a tracheal tube connector. The patient is well oxygenated but poorly ventilated, leading to progressive hypercarbia. In consequence, its use should be limited to a 45 minute period, which permits time for a definitive airway to be established.

Bibliography

Kanani M, Elliot M. *Applied Surgical Physiology Vivas*. Cambridge, Cambridge University Press; 2004.

Resuscitation Council (UK). Airway management and ventilation. In *Advanced Life Support*, 6th edn. London, Resuscitation Council (UK) Trading Ltd; 2011: Chapter 7.

Chapter 2

Breathing

Assessment

Respiratory assessment

Which basic investigations may be used in assessing respiratory function?

Following basic clinical examination of the chest during a respiratory examination, investigations may include

Non-invasive

- *Peak expiratory flow rate (PEFR)*: a bedside measure of the airway resistance and respiratory muscle function
- *Pulse oximetry*: measures arterial oxygen saturation (SaO_2) and heart rate
- *Capnography*: measures end-tidal CO_2 as a marker of ventilatory function
- *Pulmonary function tests (PFTs)*
  - Spirometry, to measure lung volumes charted on a Vitalograph®, e.g. functional expiratory volume in 1 second (FEV_1) and functional vital capacity (FVC). The FEV_1/FVC is a measure of airflow limitation and is normally >80%. Other tests include total lung capacity (TLC) and residual volume (RV). These are useful in

patients who have obstructive lung disease, e.g. asthma
and COPD

- Gas transfer, a measure of the diffusing capacity across the
  lung, e.g. transfer factor (DLco), which measures the
  transfer of low carbon monoxide concentrations in
  inspired air to haemoglobin, and transfer coefficient
  (Kco), which is the DLco corrected for alveolar volume

- *Microbiology analysis*: of sputum and retained secretions,
  including culture and cytology
- *V/Q scanning*: if pulmonary emboli are suspected
- *Echocardiography*: to assess pulmonary artery pressure and
  right heart function in cases of pulmonary hypertension and
  cor pulmonale
- *Radiology*: plain chest radiography, high-resolution CT, MRI

Invasive

- *Arterial blood gas (ABG) analysis*: directly measures
  oxygenation (PaO_2), ventilation ($PaCO_2$) and acid–base
  balance
- *Bronchoscopy*: may be flexible or rigid
- *Lung biopsy*: may be performed through a CT-guided
  approach or video-assisted thoracoscopic surgery (VATS).
  Rare cases may dictate an open operation
- *Mediastinoscopy*: performed through an incision at the root
  of the neck, permitting biopsies of regional tracheobronchial
  lymph nodes for staging pulmonary or oesophageal
  malignancy
- *Pulmonary positron emission tomography (PET)*: is a gold
  standard diagnostic procedure for evaluating the structure
  and function of pulmonary lesions, e.g. nodules or emboli

What are the applications of flexible (fibre optic) bronchoscopy?

The applications may be both diagnostic and therapeutic

- Direct visualisation of the tracheobronchial tree in cases of obstruction, e.g. retained secretions during atelectasis and aspiration of gastric contents. It may be performed through the endotracheal tube in the mechanically ventilated patient
- Biopsy for cytology or histology, which may be obtained by direct sampling or by brushings and bronchoalveolar lavage (BAL), e.g. during suspected malignancy or infection
- Difficult intubations, e.g. during insertion of double lumen tubes in thoracic or upper GI surgery for oesophagectomies
- Direct therapeutic management in the removal of foreign bodies, mucus plugs causing lobar collapse, stenting of airways in cases of acute obstruction and use of argon plasma coagulation therapy for malignant obstruction

What is the advantage of rigid over flexible bronchoscopy?

Rigid bronchoscopy permits simultaneous instrumentation due to the wider lumen. This is useful in cases of foreign body removal, e.g. coin aspiration, and it also permits suction when investigating massive haemoptysis

Which lung volumes and capacities may be measured directly and what are their normal volumes?

- *Tidal volume (TV)*: 500 ml, e.g. 7 ml/kg, represents the volume of inspired air that reaches the alveoli
- *Inspiratory reserve volume (IRV)*: 3.0 L, is the volume that can be forcibly inspired above the TV

- *Expiratory reserve volume (ERV)*: 1.3 L, is the volume that can be forcibly expired after quiet respiration

The inspiratory capacity (IC) = TV + IRV and the vital capacity (VC) = IRV + TV + ERV. Some lung volumes can only be measured by other sources

- *Residual volume (RV)*: 1.2–1.5 L, is the volume in the lungs after maximal expiration
- *Functional residual capacity (FRC)*: FRC = RV + ERV
- *Total lung volume (TLV)*: TLV = VC + RV

Define the functional residual capacity (FRC). What factors affect its volume?

The functional residual capacity is the volume of gas remaining in the lung at the end of quiet expiration. The normal range is 2.5–3.0 L.

Factors that increase the FRC

- Obstructive pulmonary diseases, e.g. asthma and COPD
- Positive end-expiratory pressure (PEEP), e.g. CPAP, which increases the intrathoracic pressure (i.e. makes it less negative)

Factors that reduce the FRC

- Age
- Obesity
- Pregnancy
- Supine position

- Factors limiting lung expansion, e.g. pleural effusion, abdominal swelling and incision, thoracic incision, restrictive lung diseases, e.g. interstitial lung disease

The FRC and RV are calculated by one of three methods, which are gas dilution, nitrogen washout or plethysmography.

How do you differentiate obstructive from restrictive diseases on spirometry?

In cases of obstructive lung disease, e.g. asthma, there is an increase in total lung capacity and residual volume due to air trapping, demonstrated by an FEV_1/FVC <80%. In restrictive lung diseases, e.g. fibrosis, there is a reduction is all lung volumes but paradoxically an increase in the FEV_1/FVC >80%.

Basic concepts

Atelectasis

What is the definition of atelectasis?

Atelectasis is defined as an absence of gas from all or part of the lung. Plain chest radiography (CXR) can demonstrate subsegmental, segmental, lobar or pulmonary collapse.

What causes atelectasis and what is the pathophysiology?

The aetiology includes

- Bronchial obstruction caused by sputum, foreign body or tumour

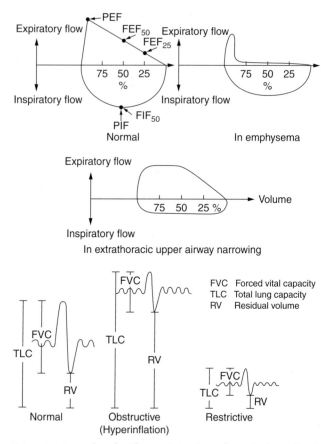

Figure 2.1 Reproduced with permission from the *Oxford Handbook of Clinical Medicine*, 8th edn. Edited by Longmore et al. (2010). Published by Oxford University Press, ISBN 9780199232178.

- Alveolar hypoventilation leading to a progressive absorption of gas and subsequent collapse of the parenchyma
- Parenchymal compression by pleural effusion or pulmonary oedema
- Inadvertent endobronchial intubation and subsequent collapse of the unventilated lung

In the case of airways obstruction there is distal gas trapping. This trapped gas is absorbed since it has a higher partial pressure than that of mixed venous blood. This leads to progressive collapse of the lung beyond the obstruction. The physiological consequence is

- V/Q mismatch and hypoxaemia
- Reduction of lung compliance and a subsequent increase in the work of breathing
- Predisposition to infection due to retention of secretions

Why might a high-inspired concentration of oxygen lead to atelectasis?

The theoretical reason lies in the higher solubility and faster absorption of oxygen compared to nitrogen. When inspiring air, the slowly absorbed nitrogen splints the airways open as oxygen is being absorbed. At a high FiO_2 this nitrogen 'splint' is theoretically reduced so that when the oxygen is absorbed, the lung unit collapses. This is called 'absorption' atelectasis.

What are the risk factors for post-operative atelectasis?

- Upper abdominal and thoracic surgery. This reduces lung expansion from pain and diaphragmatic splinting leads to retention of secretions and distal airways collapse

- Body mass index (BMI) >27
- Smoking (in the preceding 8 weeks)
- Age >59
- ASA > II
- Chronic obstructive pulmonary disease (COPD)
- Intermittent positive pressure ventilation (IPPV) > 1 day

What are the principles of post-operative atelectasis management?

- Preoperative anticipation
  - Breathing exercises before the operation may be used to improve expansion
- Intraoperative management
  - Humidification which improves mucociliary function
  - Adequate tidal volumes to ensure good expansion
  - Avoid unnecessarily high FiO_2 to prevent 'absorption' atelectasis, as evidence for its routine use is scarce and should be restricted to patients at risk of persistent hypoxaemia, e.g. obesity, COPD and those at risk of impaired tissue oxygen delivery, e.g. sickle cell disease and myocardial ischaemia
- Post-operative measures
  - Position the patient upright
  - Adequate analgesia to encourage good tidal volumes
  - Mobilise early
  - Breathing exercises, e.g. physiotherapy
  - Continuous positive airways pressure (CPAP)
  - Bronchoscopy and suction to clear mucus plugs and secretions

Also, deep breathing exercises aid lung expansion. As the lung expands, the compliance improves and through the process of radial traction, the airflow resistance falls. Both these factors contribute to a reduction in the work of breathing.

What is continuous positive airways pressure (CPAP) ventilation and what are its physiological effects on the respiratory system?

CPAP is an oxygen delivery system that relies on a closed circuit to provide positive airways pressure throughout all phases of spontaneous ventilation. The circuit can be attached to a tight-fitting mask (or tracheal tube) with a range of expiratory valves that do not open until a pressure, e.g. 2.5–10 cmH_2O, is applied. As the patient expires against valve resistance, or as gas flows into the patient during inspiration, the pressure in the airways should not drop below that indicated on the valve. It improves ventilation through

- Recruitment, e.g. opening of collapsed alveoli and prevention of their collapse on expiration
- Increasing the functional residual capacity (FRC). In the elderly and critically ill, collapse of the airways occurs close to the volume of the FRC. Alveoli recruitment increases the FRC
- Increasing lung compliance and reducing the work of breathing
- Changing the V/Q ratio, e.g. it increases, which improves oxygenation

What are the disadvantages of CPAP ventilation?
- The tight-fitting mask is uncomfortable and may be poorly tolerated, causing nasal pressure sores
- It can cause gastric dilatation due to swallowed air and regurgitation
- Barotrauma to the alveoli due to high pressure (more common in neonates)

If CPAP is not tolerated, patients develop refractory hypoxaemia, increasing respiratory rate and progressively smaller tidal volumes, and subsequent CO_2 retention.

Bronchiectasis

What do you understand by the term bronchiectasis?
This is a localised (lobar) or generalised (pulmonary) irreversible dilatation of the bronchi arising as a result of a chronic necrotising infection. There is impaired clearance of bronchial secretions. It is classed as a chronic obstructive airways disease (COAD) based on spirometry.

What causes bronchiectasis and what is the pathophysiology?
There are three overlapping pathologic forms of bronchiectasis

- *Follicular*: characterised by the loss of bronchial elastic tissue and multiple lymphoid follicles
- *Atelectatic*: a localised dilatation of the airways associated with parenchymal collapse due to a proximal airways obstruction

- *Saccular*: this exhibits patchy dilatation of the airways. In this situation there is a loss of the normal bronchial subdivisions

What is the aetiology of bronchiectasis?

A number of disease processes lead to bronchiectasis, but the basic pathogenesis involves cycles of acute and chronic inflammation accompanied by tissue damage and repair. Some of the more common causes include

- Congenital
  - *Ciliary dyskinesia*: primary ciliary dyskinesia, Kartagener's and Young's syndromes
  - *Cystic fibrosis*: the most common cause in the West
  - *Immunoglobulin deficiencies (primary)*: this is heralded by recurrent infections in infancy
- Acquired
  - *Post-infective bronchial damage*: measles, pertussis, bronchiolitis, pneumonia, adenovirus and TB
  - *Bronchial obstruction*: tumours, inhaled foreign body and extrinsic compression from lymphadenopathy
  - *Immunoglobulin deficiencies (secondary)*: AIDS
  - *Other causes*: allergic bronchopulmonary aspergillosis (ABPA), rheumatoid arthritis and ulcerative colitis

Which bacteria may colonise the airways in those with bronchiectasis?

Bacterial colonisation often involves

- *Haemophilus influenzae*
- *Streptococcus pneumoniae*

- *Staphylococcus aureus*
- *Pseudomonas aeruginosa* (in the chronically afflicted)

What complications can occur in the untreated patient with bronchiectasis?

- In the short term
  - Intermittent haemoptysis, which may be massive
  - Recurrent chest infections, lung abscesses and empyema
  - Metastatic infection, e.g. cerebral abscess
- In the long term
  - Respiratory failure due to chronic airway obstruction
  - Cor pulmonale, secondary to pulmonary hypertension
  - Secondary amyloidosis with protein A deposition

How is bronchiectasis managed?

The principles of management involve

- Management of reversible airways obstruction with bronchodilators and inhaled steroids
- Physiotherapy to encourage sputum expectoration of retained secretions and mucus drainage. Patients may also be trained to perform postural drainage techniques for use at home
- Control of infection with antibiotics, which should be prescribed according to bacterial sensitivities and local microbiology guidelines
- Management of the underlying causes, e.g. airways obstruction, cystic fibrosis
- Surgery, e.g. lobectomy, is used for localised disease in a minority of cases or to control life-threatening haemoptysis.

Severe disease sometimes requires lung transplantation, e.g. in cystic fibrosis

Pneumonia

What is the definition of pneumonia?
Pneumonia is an inflammatory condition of the lung characterised by consolidation due to exudate in the alveolar spaces.

What are the pathological types of pneumonia?
- *Lobar pneumonia*: the exudate forms directly in the bronchioles and alveoli and spills over into adjacent segments via the pore of Kohn. The consolidation is sharply confined to a particular lobe. It is typically pneumococcal in origin
- *Bronchopneumonia*: the inflammatory process starts at the bronchioles and extends into the alveoli, leading to numerous foci of consolidation. It is more common at the extremes of age
- *Interstitial pneumonia*: consists of a group of conditions characterised by chronic alveolar inflammation, which are not necessarily infective in origin and may have an immunological basis

What are the classical pathological phases of lobar pneumonia?
There are four pathologically recognised stages

- *Acute congestion (day 1–2)*: the lobe is heavy, dark and firm with inflammatory exudate and cellular infiltration, including erythrocytes
- *Red hepatisation (day 2–4)*: the lung is firm, red and consolidated. The alveolar spaces contain neutrophils, fibrin and extravasated erythrocytes
- *Grey hepatisation (day 4–8)*: the lobe is heavy, consolidated and grey. There is an extensive fibrin network with degenerating erythrocytes
- *Resolution (>day 8)*: macrophage action liquefies the exudate with fibrinolytic enzymes. Full resolution may take up to 3 weeks

How common is pneumonia in the ICU and which organisms are involved?

The type encountered in ICU is usually hospital acquired (nosocomial) occurring 48–72 hours following endotracheal intubation (or tracheostomy). It may afflict 30–40% of ventilated patients and 15–20% of the unventilated. Ventilator-associated pneumonia (VAP) may be divided into early onset (1–4 days following intubation) and late onset (beyond day 5).

Organisms involved

- *Early onset*: oropharyngeal organisms mainly, e.g. *Streptococcus pneumoniae, Staphylococcus aureus* and *Haemophilus influenzae*
- *Late onset*: usually involving gram-negative organisms, e.g. *Pseudomonas, Enterobacter, Acinetobacter*

Early-onset pneumonia carries a better prognosis than late onset, as the latter tends to be associated with multi-drug-resistant organisms, e.g. MRSA, and so is characterised by higher mortality rates. It is the leading cause of death in ICU.

What are the normal respiratory defence mechanisms against infection?

- Nasal humidification of inhaled air
- Airway mucus secretion
- Intact cough reflex
- Mucociliary action of respiratory epithelium
- Alveolar macrophages
- Secretory IgA

What are the risk factors for nosocomial pneumonia in the intubated patient?

- Loss of the anatomic barriers due to instrumentation. Organisms can enter the lower respiratory tract when the epiglottis and glottis are breached by the endotracheal tube
- Impaired cough reflex as the endotracheal tube opens the glottis
- Re-intubation
- Colonisation of other instruments, e.g. tubing in the ventilator circuit and Y-connectors for tubing
- Aspiration of gastric contents which may be colonised by bacteria
- Prone positioning predisposes to aspiration
- Epithelial trauma to the airway, e.g. by suction devices
- Cross-colonisation from staff and other patients

- Generalised debilitating or chronic illness, e.g. malignancy, diabetes mellitus, burns, general trauma and uraemia

Which factors predispose the stomach to bacterial colonisation?

The risk of bacterial colonisation increases when the gastric pH > 4.0, and this can increase the risk of acquiring pneumonia

- Use of H-blockers and PPIs to prevent stress ulceration (the risk of colonisation is reduced if sucralfate is preferentially used)
- Continuous gastric feeding
- Chronic atrophic gastritis leading to achlorhydria

How is pneumonia recognised in the ICU setting?

The gold standard for the diagnosis of pneumonia in the ICU is direct biopsy of suspected lung tissue, but this is not ideal as it usually occurs at post-mortem. Many of the clinical features are common to a number of conditions, e.g. atelectasis and include

- Clinical
  - Clinical signs on examination
  - Pyrexia $>38.3°C$
  - Leucocytosis $>12 \times 10^9$/ml
  - Purulent tracheobronchial secretions
- Radiological
  - New and persistent pulmonary infiltrates on plain chest radiography

- Microbiological
    - Blood and pleural fluid
    - Gram staining and cultures of tracheal secretions
- Bronchoscopic
    - Brushings
    - Bronchoalveolar lavage (BAL)
- Non-bronchoscopic
    - Transthoracic needle biopsy
    - Open/VATS lung biopsy

How can pneumonia be prevented?

Prevention is always more effective than prolonged antibiotic treatment. This involves

- Protective isolation of high-risk patients
- Control of cross-infection by staff, e.g. effective hand-washing
- Oral hygiene care
- Suctioning of subglottic secretions
- Intermittent and not continuous enteral feeding
- Controlled use of antibiotics to prevent multi-drug resistance, e.g. super-infection
- Use of sucralfate for stress ulcer prophylaxis
- Decreasing the number of times that the ventilator circuit is broken by connections

What are the complications of bacterial pneumonia in critical care?

Complications include

- *Respiratory failure*: Type I respiratory failure is common, requiring high-flow oxygen and repeated ABGs to check for PaO_2 and $PaCO_2$ for worsening acidosis
- *Pleuritis*: leading to pleural effusions and healing with extensive pleural adhesions
- *Pleural effusion*: an accumulation of fluid in the pleural space requiring aspiration if small and tube drainage if large
- *Empyema*: this is a loculated collection of pus in the pleural cavity. It generates recurrent fevers in a resolving pneumonia requiring tube drainage before a thick fibrinous cortex develops
- *Lung abscess*: a cavitating area of suppurative infection in lung parenchyma. This can erode to form a bronchopleural fistula and empyema
- *Metastatic abscesses*: spread to distant sites can form cerebral abscesses
- *Septicaemia*: in any form, and can cause metastatic spread, e.g. infective endocarditis, meningitis and hypotension, and atrial fibrillation may develop (driven by the sepsis)

Pneumothorax

What types of pneumothorax are there and what are their identifying features?

There are three types of pneumothorax

- *Simple pneumothorax*: where there is air in the pleural space, but no cardiovascular compromise

- *Tension pneumothorax*: there is a one-way valve effect that allows air to enter the pleural space, but not to leave it. Mediastinal shift and compression from the air in the pleural space displaces the heart and great vessels, producing deleterious cardiorespiratory embarrassment and shock
- *Open pneumothorax (the 'sucking chest wound')*: an open defect in the thoracic wall draws in air during the respiratory cycle, leading to tension pneumothorax

Note that a simple pneumothorax, if left unmanaged, may lead to a tension pneumothorax when it becomes large enough to cause mediastinal shift.

What are the causes of pneumothoraces?
- Primary
  - *Spontaneous*: following the rupture of apical blebs of unknown origin
- Secondary
  - *Spontaneous*: pre-existing lung disease including asthma, cystic fibrosis and bullous disease in COPD
  - *Traumatic*: due to both blunt and penetrating trauma
  - *Iatrogenic*: following pleural aspiration, central line insertion, oesophagoscopy and barotrauma from IPPV

What are the signs on clinical examination?
For a simple pneumothorax

- Ipsilateral reduction of chest wall movements
- Increased resonance on percussion
- Reduced breath sounds on the affected side

- Tachypnoea
- Tachycardia (a non-specific sign)
- Hypoxia
- Occasionally the presence of subcutaneous emphysema

With a tension pneumothorax the above signs exist together with

- Hypotension
- Elevated JVP
- Cyanosis despite tachypnoea
- Pulsus paradoxus
- Tracheal deviation indicating mediastinal shift to the opposite side (a late sign indicating impending doom)
- Reduced GCS
- Rapid clinical deterioration leading to respiratory arrest

How may pneumothorax be recognised in the mechanically ventilated patient?

- Sudden increase in the inflation pressure
- Sudden and unexplained hypoxia
- Development of new cardiac arrhythmia, e.g. atrial fibrillation
- Sudden hypotension
- Rising JVP

How is the diagnosis of pneumothorax confirmed?

For simple pneumothoraces an erect CXR during expiration confirms the diagnosis. A tension pneumothorax is a clinical diagnosis that must be managed by life-saving needle decompression. Only then should a CXR be ordered.

How is pneumothorax managed?

All types require the airway to be secured and administration of 100% oxygen by a non-re-breath face mask during ABCDE assessment and the ordering of ABGs and CXRs.

- *Simple pneumothoraces*: treatment depends on the presence (or absence) of breathlessness, size of air (<2 cm vs. >2 cm) on CXR and age of the patient (<50 vs. >50), which determines pleural aspiration or chest drainage
- *Tension pneumothoraces*: managed by emergency needle decompression, and chest tube thoracostomy is required once the tension has been converted to a simple pneumothorax. This also drains blood in traumatic cases
- *Open pneumothorax*: an occlusive dressing is applied to the surface of the wound, being taped down on three sides. This acts as a one-way valve allowing air to escape on expiration and preventing air entry on inspiration

Recurrent cases of spontaneous pneumothoraces may be managed by open or thoracoscopic pleurectomy and pleurodesis. By stripping the parietal pleura, adhesions form between the lung and chest wall preventing further collapse.

How is emergency decompression of a tension pneumothorax carried out?

- A large bore (14- or 16-gauge) cannula is inserted into the 2nd intercostal space in the mid-clavicular line. It must pass along the superior border of the 3rd rib to prevent injury to the neurovascular bundle of the 2nd rib

- The correct position is confirmed by the presence of the hissing sound of escaping air
- A chest drain is prepared for definitive management

Complex concepts

Acute respiratory distress syndrome (ARDS)

What is the definition of lung compliance?

Lung compliance is the change in lung volume per unit change in pressure, e.g. the ease with which the lung inflates. The greater the compliance, the greater the volume increase for a particular change in pressure. The overall compliance of the lung is 200 ml/cmH$_2$O.

What is lung surfactant composed of and what purpose does it serve?

Surfactant is a phospholipid mixture of dipalmitoylphosphatidylcholine, cholesterol, lipids and other proteins. It is produced by Type II pneumocytes and acts to reduce the surface tension of fluid lining the alveoli. This increases the compliance according to Laplace's law, i.e. a smaller transpulmonary pressure is required to overcome the surface tension when inflating the alveolus. Consequently

- The work of breathing is reduced

- Smaller alveoli are stabilised, preventing their collapse during deflation and subsequent atelectasis
- Fluid is optimised, e.g. keeps them relatively dry by reducing transudation of fluid from the interstitium

What is the definition of ARDS?

ARDS is a syndrome of acute respiratory failure and persistent inflammatory disease of the lungs. Associative signs include reduced lung compliance, hypoxaemia, which is refractory to oxygen therapy, and the formation of non-cardiogenic pulmonary oedema. The changes are seen as

- Diffuse bilateral pulmonary infiltrates seen on chest radiography, not fully explained by effusions, fluid overload or lung collapse
- Pulmonary artery capillary wedge pressure (PACWP) of <18 mmHg, excludes a cardiac cause due to no atrial hypertension
- PaO_2/FiO_2 ratio of <26.6 kPa (200 mmHg)

How does it relate to acute lung injury (ALI) and the systemic inflammatory response syndrome (SIRS)?

ALI comprises a number of non-specific pathological changes in the lung parenchyma in response to a specific insult. These changes are like that of ARDS but less severe, e.g. PaO_2/FiO_2 is <40 kPa (300 mmHg). ARDS is at the extreme end of the spectrum of ALI and is the respiratory component of SIRS associated with multi-organ dysfunction.

What are the causes of ARDS?

The triggering factors can be organised into direct and indirect insults to the lung

- Direct insults
  - Pneumonia
  - Aspiration
  - Pulmonary contusion
  - Fat emboli
  - Near-drowning
  - Inhalational injury, e.g. smoke
  - Reperfusion pulmonary oedema
- Indirect insults
  - Severe sepsis and evidence of organ hypoperfusion, e.g. oliguria, lactic acidosis, reduced GCS
  - Severe trauma, including hypovolaemic shock
  - Massive transfusion
  - Drug overdose
  - Disseminated intravascular coagulation (DIC)
  - Acute pancreatitis
  - Cardiopulmonary bypass
  - Pregnancy-related ARDS

Discuss the process that leads to its effects on the lung

The pathophysiological changes may be seen in the following flow diagram

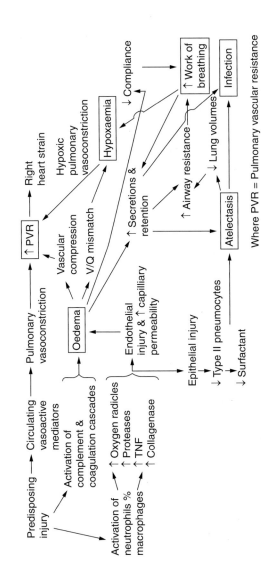

Figure 2.2

The histopathological changes are divided into a number of discrete phases that can take less than 24 hours to establish

- Inflammatory phase (initial) 3–5 days
    - Activated neutrophils and macrophages release several mediators such as oxygen-free radicals, proteases, prostaglandins, tumour necrosis factor (TNF) and collagenases
    - Local activation of the complement and coagulation cascades
    - Endothelial injury leads to increased capillary permeability and the formation of pulmonary oedema
    - Epithelial injury manifests as a decrease of Type II pneumocytes, reducing surfactant production
- Proliferative phase (sub-acute) 5–10 days
    - Increased alveolar dead space
    - Interstitial fibrosis and proliferation of Type II alveolar cells
    - Increase in the local fibroblast population
- Progressive phase (chronic) 14–n days
    - Increase in dead space ventilation
    - Extensive pulmonary fibrosis
    - Obliteration of normal alveolar architecture
    - Widespread emphysema and discrete bullae

Consequently, there are a number of physiological changes in the lung

- Oedema and decreased lung volume leads to a fall in lung compliance, which increases the work of breathing

- Increased secretions and their retention give rise to local atelectasis and a reduction of the FRC
- Worsening shunt and V/Q mismatch leading to hypoxaemia and respiratory failure
- Pulmonary vascular resistance increases due to the oedema compressing the vessels, and by hypoxic pulmonary vasoconstriction occurring as a defence mechanism in order to improve the V/Q
- Atelectasis, endothelial and epithelial injury predisposes to infection
- Pulmonary hypertension increases the work of the right side of the heart, and can lead to right heart dysfunction
- Progressive interstitial fibrosis may persist even after the patient has recovered

What are the principles of management?

The principles of management lie in a number of supportive measures following ABCDE assessment

- Management of the initial predisposing insult
- Adequate nutritional support, e.g. during severe sepsis and trauma
- Mechanical ventilation to improve oxygenation and elimination of CO_2. High levels of positive end-expiratory pressure (PEEP), e.g. 10–20 cmH$_2$O, may be used to hold open the alveoli throughout the whole respiratory cycle, but this risks barotrauma to the lung
- Small tidal volumes have been shown to improve outcome. This leads to a permanent hypercarbia, e.g. $PaCO_2$ >6.7 kPa, which is usually well tolerated

- Changing, e.g. inverting, the usual inspiratory:expiratory (I:E) ratio of 1:2. The length of the inspiratory phase is increased to improve oxygenation of the small obstructed airways
- Prone positioning during intermittent positive pressure ventilation (IPPV) redistributes secretions, as dependent lung regions are preferentially infiltrated, consolidated or collapsed. This alters the V/Q and improves oxygenation
- Strict control of fluid resuscitation to prevent worsening pulmonary oedema
- Inhaled nitric oxide and aerosolised epoprostenol induces localised pulmonary vasodilatation, which reduces pulmonary hypertension and transiently increases oxygenation to improve the V/Q. The impact on survival is equivocal

What is the prognosis?

The outcome is poor as mortality ranges from 30 to 60%. ARDS in the presence of sepsis has the poorest outcome and mortality increases to 90%.

What is the mechanism of action of nitric oxide?

Nitric oxide (NO) is an endothelium-derived relaxing factor (EDRF) which activates the cytoplasmic enzyme guanylyl cyclase. This increases the intracellular cyclic guanosine monophosphate (cGMP) levels, which stimulates a cGMP-dependent protein kinase. The activated protein kinase stimulates the phosphorylation of key proteins in a pathway that leads to a relaxation of vascular smooth muscle cells.

Flail chest

What are the defining features of a flail chest injury?
A flail chest occurs when there are three or more ribs fractured at two or more places on the rib shaft. This gives rise to an area of the chest wall that has lost bony continuity with the rest of the rib cage and has the potential to move autonomously during the respiratory cycle.

How much blood may be lost from a single rib fracture?
A rib fracture may be associated with the loss of 150 ml of blood

What are the implications of finding a flail segment?
- *Severity marker*: it takes a lot of kinetic energy to fracture several ribs at once owing to their elastic properties, indicating a probable violent mechanism of injury
- *Co-existing injuries*: other thoracic injuries such as pulmonary contusion, haemothorax, pneumothorax, blunt cardiac trauma or diaphragmatic rupture are highly probable
- *Early complications*: if severe enough, flail chest injuries may lead to respiratory failure in the absence of other associated thoracic injuries
- *Late complications*: may include septicaemia due to retained secretions, atelectasis and pneumonia if not adequately treated

What are the pathophysiological changes to the respiratory system that can occur with flail chest injury?
- The flail segment exhibits paradoxical motion during the respiratory cycle, i.e. it moves inwards during inspiration

because it is drawn in by the increasingly negative intrapleural pressure. This reduces the tidal volume
- Pain from the injury also reduces the tidal volume
- Reduced tidal volumes and an inefficient cough mechanism due to pain leads to retention of secretions
- Subsequent atelectasis causes V/Q mismatching that can lead to Type I respiratory failure
- A predisposition to Type II respiratory failure exists following the loss of the normal chest wall mechanical apparatus
- Underlying pulmonary contusion can exacerbate all of these effects

What are the principles of management of flail chest injury?
This injury must be managed in the context of the ATLS® protocol

- Management of the flail segment itself
- Identification of injuries to the underlying thoracic organs
- Preventing complications such as atelectasis and pneumonia

The vast majority of patients may be conservatively managed and surgical intervention in the form of chest wall fixation is rarely required

- Humidified oxygen
- Adequate analgesia for pain relief, which helps to improve respiratory physiology and permit effective physiotherapy
- Intubation and mechanical ventilation in cases of worsening fatigue and respiratory failure

- Minitracheostomy, which can help to clear secretions and avert mechanical ventilation in the progressively decompensating patient

How may pain relief be achieved in these cases?

Analgesia is titrated to clinical response and includes paracetamol, NSAIDs and opiates that may be given enterally or parenterally. A commonly used parenteral route is thoracic epidural anaesthesia and the level of the block extends to T4.

What is a sucking chest wound and how may it be immediately managed in the emergency setting?

A sucking chest wound occurs when the diameter of an open chest wall defect is greater than two-thirds the diameter of the trachea. Consequently, on inspiration, air preferentially enters the chest cavity through the open wound and does not escape on expiration. It therefore leads to a rapidly developing tension pneumothorax. It is managed by applying an occlusive dressing that is covered on three sides. This acts as a flutter valve, preventing air entering on inspiration and permitting air to escape on expiration.

Pulmonary thromboembolism (PE)

What are the risk factors for deep venous thrombosis (DVT) and subsequent pulmonary embolism (PE)?

- Surgical
  - Neurosurgery, e.g. due to controversies in LMWH thromboprophylaxis

- Major abdominal or pelvic surgery
- Recent hip or knee surgery
- Caesarean section
- Venous stasis from immobilisation, e.g. prolonged post-operative bed rest
- General medical illness
  - Age
  - Malignancy
  - Dehydration, e.g. nephrotic syndrome
  - Severe sepsis
  - Heart disease, e.g. cardiac failure, recent myocardial infarction
  - Cerebral vascular stroke
  - Hypertension
  - COPD
  - Inflammatory bowel disease
  - Obesity
  - Polycythaemia
- Trauma
  - Lower limb injury
  - Spinal cord injury
- Haematological propensity, e.g. thrombophilias
  - Protein C or Protein S deficiencies
  - Antithrombin III deficiency
  - Factor V Leiden deficiency
  - Antiphospholipid antibodies
  - Homocysteinaemia
  - Prothrombin gene variant

- Endocrine
  - Hormone replacement therapy (HRT)
  - Oral contraceptive pill (OCP)
- Vascular
  - Previous venous thromboembolism
  - Varicose veins

In any particular patient the risk factors are often multiple and DVTs can occur in 25–50% of surgical patients.

What is a DVT and where do they commonly form?
This is a lesion that usually occurs in normal vessels, contrasting arterial thrombosis, in the deep veins of the calf and venous plexus in the soleus muscle. It specifically forms around the valves as red thrombi, consisting of erythrocytes and fibrin. Such thrombi may occur more *proximally* in the external and common iliac veins, propagating proximally to the inferior vena cava and increasing the risk of embolisation to pulmonary vessels. They may also form in the right atrium, and act as a source of pulmonary emboli in atrial fibrillation.

How may a DVT present?
- It may be asymptomatic but tenderness at the calf is the usual painful symptom
- *Phlegmasia cerulean dolens*: an acutely ischaemic and cyanotic leg following a massive ileo-femoral venous thrombosis

- *Phlegmasia alba dolens*: an acutely ischaemic and swollen white leg following a massive ileo-femoral DVT (and arterial spasm)
- Pulmonary embolism

What is the pathophysiology of a PE?

There is pulmonary artery obstruction as the embolus impacts in a vascular branch beyond the right ventricular outflow tract. Activated platelets in the thrombus release vasoactive mediators, which increase pulmonary vascular resistance and right ventricular afterload. This produces ventricular strain and a resultant tachycardia. Decreased pulmonary blood flow causes a V/Q mismatch and increased physiological dead space, and the circulating mediators can cause bronchospasm. Consequently, there is hypoxia, hypocarbia and tachypnoea.

How may a PE present?

PE may present in a number of ways depending on size, site, number and acuteness of the event

- Small PEs (and medium PEs)
  - Dypsnoea
  - Pleuritic chest pain
  - Tachypnoea
  - Tachycardia
  - Pleural rub
  - Pleural effusion, which will be exudative in nature due to being blood stained
  - Haemoptysis, due to pulmonary infarction

- Large PEs (in addition to the above)
  - Severe central chest pain
  - Shock, due to obstruction of right ventricular outflow. This results in a low cardiac index manifested as cool, pale peripheries, central cyanosis and systemic hypotension
  - Signs of right ventricular afterload, evidenced by a wide splitting heart sound, a loud pulmonary component, accentuation of the 3rd or 4th heart sounds, functional tricuspid regurgitation (a raised JVP) and a right ventricular heave
  - Sudden cardiac death or cardiac arrest, most probably pulseless electrical activity (PEA)

Chronic, multiple emboli can present with secondary pulmonary hypertension and cor pulmonale. Paradoxical embolisation can occur through a patent foramen ovale (PFO), resulting in systemic embolisation.

List the investigations that can be used to make a diagnosis of PE and DVT

In both pathological processes ABCDE assessment is required, but in the case of a PE

- ECG
- CXR, which can exclude differential diagnoses
- ABG analysis, demonstrating a V/Q mismatch seen as hypoxia and hypocarbia
- Plasma D-dimer levels, usually extremely elevated but is a non-specific test in the chronically sick patient

- V/Q scan, inconclusive in co-existent chronic lung disease, e.g. COPD
- Spiral CT and CT pulmonary angiography (CTPA)
- Pulmonary angiography is the gold standard and is useful if non-invasive methods are equivocal

In most instances, if a high index of clinical suspicion exists of an acute PE and the patient has a likely 2-level PE Wells score, guidelines suggest

- CTPA, or commence immediate anticoagulant therapy followed by a CTPA if one cannot be carried out immediately
- Compression ultrasonography (CUS) if CTPA is negative and a DVT is suspected
- V/Q single photon emission computed tomography (V/Q SPECT) scan or V/Q planar scan, as an alternative to CTPA, if patients have allergies to contrast media or severe renal impairment. And, if not available, commence immediate anticoagulation

In cases of a suspected DVT and the patient has a likely 2-level DVT Wells score, guidelines suggest

- CUS of a proximal leg vein <4 hours and, if negative or it cannot be carried out in <4 hours, a D-dimer and immediate anticoagulation until one can be arranged in <24 hours

What are the most common ECG changes in acute PEs and why do these changes occur?
The most common ECG change is sinus tachycardia and tall P-waves in lead II, right axis deviation, right bundle branch

block and T-wave inversion in the anterior leads, indicating right ventricular strain. This may represent reciprocal changes arising from inferior or posterior ischaemia, when an overloaded right ventricle compresses the right coronary artery.

What is a D-dimer and how useful a diagnostic investigation is this?

A D-dimer is a fibrin degradation product formed by the action of plasmin on the fibrin clot. It may be measured by a latex agglutination test or enzyme-linked immunosorbent assay (ELISA). It misses 10% of those with a PE.

What is the treatment of PEs and DVTs?

- Pharmacological
  - *LMWH*: e.g. dalteparin or fundaparinux sodium, adjusting the dose based on anti-Xa assays in both PE and *proximal* DVT. In established renal failure, eGFR $<30 \text{ ml/min}/1.73 \text{ m}^2$ or patients at risk of a bleeding diathesis commence unfractionated heparin, adjusting doses according to the APTT. This should be continued for 5 days
  - *Vitamin K antagonist (VKA)*: e.g. warfarin, commenced simultaneously to LMWH treatment until the INR is >2 for 24 h. Then the LMWH is stopped. This should be continued for 3 months and then reviewed by a haematologist
  - *Catheter-directed thrombolysis*: this may be considered in *proximal* DVTs if symptoms are <14 days, good

functional status, life expectancy >1 year and a low risk of
bleeding
- *Systemic thrombolysis*: e.g. using streptokinase or
  urokinase. This should be considered in patients with an
  acute PE and haemodynamic instability, which may be
  infused directly in the pulmonary artery
- Interventional radiology
  - *Pulmonary catheterisation*: this can be performed in
    patients with an acute PE and haemodynamic instability if
    thrombolysis is contraindicated due to high risk of
    haemorrhage
- Surgical
  - *Embolectomy*: this can be performed as an open
    technique in critically sick patients if thrombolysis is
    contraindicated, or if pulmonary catheterisation fails

During cardiopulmonary resuscitation, a precordial thump
may help to dislodge an obstructing mass and thrombolysis is
advocated. However, mortality in this category of patients can
be >65%.

How can PEs and DVTs be prevented?
- Stop procoagulant drugs 4 weeks preoperatively, e.g. OCP
- Thromboembolic deterrent stockings (TEDS)
- Perioperative use of LMWH, e.g. 5000 U dalteparin SC in
  low-risk patients, or unfractionated heparin, e.g. as an
  infusion in high-risk patients, ensuring the $APPT_r$ is
  1.5–2.5
- Intermittent pneumatic compression

- Inferior vena cava devices, e.g. umbrella filters to prevent recurrent emboli
- Early mobilisation

Respiratory failure

What is the normal range for the PaO_2 and $PaCO_2$ in an individual breathing air at sea level?

The normal ranges are $PaO_2 = 10.6$–13.3 kPa and $PaCO_2 = 4.7$–6.0 kPa.

Why is ventilatory function best assessed by measuring the $PaCO_2$?

Alveolar ventilation (VA) is the volume of air which enters the alveoli each minute. Since all of the CO_2 produced by the body is excreted by exhalation during the process of alveolar ventilation

$PaCO_2 \times VA$ = volume of CO_2 exhaled in 1 minute

$(PaCO_2 \propto 1/VA)$

It can be seen that measuring the CO_2 is key to assessing ventilation.

What is the definition of respiratory failure?

This is a failure of oxygenation manifested by a PaO_2 of <8 kPa owing to inadequate pulmonary gas exchange. It may also occur in the context of inadequate ventilation and subsequent CO_2 retention, e.g. $PaCO_2 > 6.7$ kPa. The definition, therefore, depends on ABG analysis, but early recognition can be made on clinical suspicion.

How may respiratory failure be classified?

Respiratory failure is classified as types I and II and mixed depending on the CO_2

- *Type I (hypoxaemic) failure*: PaO_2 <8 kPa and a normal or reduced $PaCO_2$ <6.7 kPa. It is due primarily to a V/Q mismatch, right to left shunting of blood (a pure mismatch when the V/Q is 0). There is an initial elevation of the $PaCO_2$ stimulating the central chemoreceptors that are sensitive to a local increase in the H^+ formed when CO_2 dissolves in CSF. The resulting stimulation of ventilation expels CO_2, keeping the level in the normal range (or below it). Due to the plateau of the sigmoidal O_2 dissociation curve, increasing the ventilation raises the PaO_2 very little. The outcome is therefore persisting hypoxaemia in the face of a normal or reduced $PaCO_2$ and tachypnoea
- *Type II (ventilatory) failure*: PaO_2 <8 kPa and $PaCO_2$ >6.7 kPa. It is characterised by alveolar hypoventilation leading to progressive hypercarbia ± V/Q mismatch. There is no compensatory increase in the ventilation, because of respiratory dysfunction and no subsequent compensation for a chronically elevated $PaCO_2$ as in COPD
- *Mixed defect*: the most common defect in the practical setting. A classic example is with any cause of a Type I defect where the patient develops exhaustion, producing a progressive and pre-terminal hypercarbia

Why should respiratory failure be classified?

The main purpose of classification lies in the practical use of oxygen as the therapeutic tool. In cases of chronic CO_2

retention, oxygen has to be used with caution (*see* Chapter 1, Oxygen: Therapy).

Give some examples of the different causes of respiratory failure

Type I

- Shunt
  - Intracardiac, e.g. congenital cyanotic heart disease, Eisenmenger's syndrome
- V/Q mismatch
  - Pneumonia, and shunting may occur at some lung units that are not being ventilated owing to inflammatory exudate
  - Pneumothorax
  - Pulmonary embolism
  - Pulmonary oedema, e.g. cardiac failure, ARDS
  - Bronchiectasis, severe asthma
  - Fibrosing alveolitis

Type II

- Lung parenchymal lesions
  - COPD, life-threatening asthma, pneumonia, pulmonary fibrosis, obstructive sleep apnoea
- Cerebral lesions
  - Head injury, brainstem stroke, sedative drugs, e.g. barbiturates
- Neuromuscular lesions

- High cervical trauma, poliomyelitis, diaphragmatic paralysis, motor neurone disease (MND), Guillan-Barré syndrome (GBS), exhaustion, e.g. asthma
- Thoracic cage lesions
  - Flail chest injury, kyphoscoliosis

Outline the principles of management of respiratory failure
The basic principles are ABCDE assessment, including

- Adequate oxygenation, preferably humidified, which should be controlled in cases of COPD, e.g. FiO_2 24%, but, nevertheless, hypoxia should not be left untreated
- Adequate ventilation, may need non-IPPV, e.g. CPAP, or intubation and IPPV depending on the clinical impression and serial ABG analysis
- Antibiotic treatment if the underlying process is infective, which is empirical in the emergency setting
- Treatment of the underlying cause, e.g. bronchodilators and steroids in asthma, and management of pain

Procedures

Chest drains: the surgical way

What is the purpose of a chest drain?
This is a therapeutic procedure enabling drainage of air and fluid, e.g. effusions, blood, pus and lymph, from the pleural space to enable lung re-expansion and restoration of normal negative intrapleural pressure and respiratory function. It can

be used as a diagnostic procedure to permit microbiological analysis of fluid. A chest drain is inserted in these conditions

- Pneumothorax, e.g. simple and tension (after initial needle decompression)
- Haemothorax
- Chylothorax
- Pleural effusion, e.g. transudate, exudate
- Empyema
- Post-operative cardiac, thoracic and oesophagectomy surgery

The majority are inserted intraoperatively under direct vision. If inserted on the ward, e.g. due to a tension pneumothorax, it should be placed according to both British Thoracic Society (BTS) guidelines and the ATLS® protocol. Due to the risks of surgical chest drains, all operators should be adequately trained.

What are the pre-procedure checks required for a safe insertion?

All indications for a surgical chest drain require ABCDE assessment, reviewing of laboratory and radiological investigations and assembly of all required equipment. The exception is a tension pneumothorax, i.e. immediate needle decompression

- Laboratory
  - *Prothrombin time (PT)*: it is good medical practice to check this, e.g. in patients on warfarin anticoagulation,

despite there being no evidence that deranged clotting exacerbates post-procedure bleeding

- *Platelet count*: it is prudent to check this in patients at risk of prolonged bleeding due to haematological diseases, e.g. haemophilia
- Radiological
  - *CXR*: this is mandatory due to the risk of iatrogenic injury to the liver and spleen, traumatising lung densely adherent to the chest wall, e.g. in a haemothorax, which is an absolute contraindication, and assessing differential diagnoses

Written informed consent from the patient should be obtained to both the chest drain and appropriate local anaesthetic (and light sedation if necessary). Patients should be transferred to an HDU bed to permit cardiorespiratory monitoring throughout the procedure.

List the equipment needed and outline the steps for insertion

A surgical chest drain usually comes in a sterile pack and includes sterile drapes, gauze swabs, selection of needles, scalpel and blade, Robert's forceps (curved clamps) and a basic surgical tray. Other pieces include sterile gloves and gown, antiseptic solution, local anaesthetic, suture, chest drain, connecting tubing, closed drainage system (including sterile water if underwater seal is being used) and dressings all opened in an aseptic non-touch sterile technique.

- *Positioning*: the patient is positioned supine, the arm on the side of insertion is abducted and the hand placed under the occiput
- *Marking*: a rib overlying the insertion point is marked, e.g. 5th intercostal space in the mid-axillary line, but clinical judgement based on reviewing the CXR dictates the insertion point
- *Prep. and drape*: following scrubbing and gowning, the skin is cleaned from clavicle to pelvis using Betadine® and the patient is draped exposing the designated area
- *Infiltration of local anaesthetic (LA)*: e.g. 2 ml 1% lignocaine (lidocaine) is used to make a small wheal over the skin using an orange needle before 10–15 ml is used to progressively infiltrate the subcutaneous layers using a white needle. It is advanced over the top of the rib to prevent injury to the neurovascular bundle in the subcostal grove of the overlying rib. More can be infiltrated before the parietal pleura is breached
- *Incision*: a 2–3 cm transverse stab incision is made using a size 11 blade overlying the insertion site
- *Blunt dissection*: a Robert's clamp is used to make a path through the chest wall opening up muscle fibres down to the parietal pleura. Sometimes a finger is used to widen the tract. To confirm correct positioning, a needle and syringe is used to aspirate air or fluid before puncturing the pleura using the clamp. Once inside, a finger is used to explore the thoracic cavity, clearing any adhesions
- *Securing the incision*: before inserting the drain, two 0 silk sutures are placed, e.g. a mattress suture across the incision,

to assist closure of the incision once the drain is removed and a stay suture to secure the drain

- *Insertion*: an appropriately sized tube, e.g. 24-Fr for pneumothoraces or 32-Fr for haemothoraces, is clamped at the tip using the Robert's forceps and it is pushed to the desired length through the tract, being guided apically to drain air or basally to drain fluid. Once inside, the tube is secured and a dressing is applied
- *Closed system drainage*: the end of the tube is connected to an underwater drainage system to permit one directional flow. Check for air bubbling in the water. It should be held below the level of the patient and the tube end no more than 5 cm below the water line (to prevent increased resistance to air evacuation) to enable swing in respiration to be evaluated

Following successful insertion, a CXR should be ordered to check for lung re-expansion and an ABG conducted to analyse PaO_2 and $PaCO_2$. In the correct clinical setting, e.g. thoracic ward, suction can be applied to aid lung re-expansion.

What are the complications of chest drain insertion?
The complications include

- Early
  - Malpositioning if inserted too far so that it coils and kinks
  - Haemothorax from neurovascular bundle trauma, pulmonary vascular laceration
  - Pulmonary damage due to iatrogenic laceration and contusion
  - Abdominal injury to bowel, liver and spleen

- Late
  - Blocked drain if clots form in the drain from haemothoraces
  - Pneumothorax if a tension develops following removal
  - Pleural air leak due to the tube being inserted into the lung parenchyma

What are the indications for removal of the drain?
- Re-expansion has been successful and demonstrated on CXR
- The drain is no longer functioning
- Air and fluid have ceased to drain, e.g. no further respiratory swing on the drain, cessation of bubbling seen when suction is applied (suggesting that a parenchymal air leak has sealed)

Bibliography

American College of Surgeons. Thoracic trauma. In *Advanced Trauma Life Support® (ATLS®)*, 9th edn. Chicago, IL, American College of Surgeons; 2012: Chapter 4.

Koenig SM, Truwit JD. Ventilator-associated pneumonia: diagnosis, treatment, and prevention. *Clinical Microbiology Reviews.* 2006;19(4): 637–57.

NICE Clinical Guideline 144. Venous thromboembolic diseases: the management of venous thromboembolic diseases and the role of thrombophilia testing. *National Institute for Health and Clinical Excellence (NICE)*. 2012;144: 1–40.

SIGN Clinical Guideline 77. Postoperative management in adults: a practical guide to postoperative care for clinical staff. Chapter 4 respiratory management. *Scottish Intercollegiate Guidelines Network (SIGN)*. 2004;77: 20–7.

Chapter 3

Circulation

Assessment

Cardiac assessment

Which basic investigations may be used in assessing cardiovascular function?

Following basic clinical examination of the praecordium during a cardiovascular examination, investigations may include

Non-invasive

- *Pulse*: this is a clinical assessment of rate and rhythm, e.g. radial artery, and volume and character, e.g. carotid artery
- *Non-invasive blood pressure (NIBP)*: this employs a sphygmomanometer, e.g. manual measurement, or a Dinamap®, e.g. automated monitoring. The Dinamap® can measure absolute values, mean and pulse pressure, but mercury measurement is more accurate
- *Electrocardiograph (ECG)*: measures the rate, rhythm, intervals, axis and waveforms
- *Transthoracic echocardiography (TTE)*: measures systolic function, cardiac filling, valve function general morphology and blood flow

- *Radiology*: plain chest radiography (cardiothoracic ratio), CT, MRI

Other non-invasive assessments include the clinical evaluation of GCS, as a marker of cerebral perfusion, capillary refill time and urine output as markers of cardiac index (CI) and organ function, e.g. renal function.

Invasive

- *Intra-arterial blood pressure (IABP)*: e.g. radial arterial line, exhibits a continuous arterial waveform and beat to beat variation
- *Central venous catheter (CVC)*: e.g. internal jugular vein, measures the central venous pressure (CVP) or its response to fluid challenges and inotropes. The waveform may be continuously displayed
- *Pulmonary artery flotation catheter (PAFC)*: provides both direct and derived measures of left heart function, e.g. cardiac output. It also measures systemic and pulmonary vascular resistance, e.g. pulmonary artery capillary wedge pressure (PACWP), oxygen delivery, SaO_2 and demand
- *Transoesophageal echocardiography (TOE [TEE])*: Gives a more detailed picture of the left heart and thoracic aorta than transthoracic echocardiography
- *Cardiac catheterisation and coronary angiography*: is the gold standard diagnostic procedure regarding the structure and function of the heart

Other invasive assessments of cardiac index and peripheral organ perfusion include

- *Arterial blood gases (ABGs)*: to assess the acidosis and base excess associated with anaerobic metabolism following poor tissue perfusion
- *Biochemistry*: rising serum lactate levels indicate a poor cardiac index
- *Gastric tonometry*: adequacy of splanchnic perfusion is estimated from gastric intramucosal pH measurements using a gastric probe. The gut is the first organ system to reflect a poor peripheral perfusion
- *Arteriovenous oxygen difference (a–vO$_2$)*: oxygen extraction is increased in cases of poor organ perfusion due to relative stagnation

Blood pressure monitoring

Define the blood pressure

Blood pressure (BP) is the product of the cardiac output (CO) and the systemic vascular resistance (SVR). The CO is the product of the heart rate (HR) and stroke volume (SV) and has a resting value of 5–6 L min^{-1}.

How can blood pressure be monitored?

Blood pressure can be measured non-invasively (NIBP), e.g. sphygmomanometer, or invasively by direct cannulation of a peripheral artery, e.g. invasive arterial blood pressure monitoring (*see* Arterial Lines: Intra-Arterial Blood Pressure Monitoring). The latter provides a continuous waveform trace after attachment to an electronic pressure transducer.

How does invasive monitoring compare to non-invasive monitoring?

Invasive blood pressure monitoring, e.g. radial lines measure systolic BP 5 mmHg higher and diastolic BP 8 mmHg lower than non-invasive blood pressure measurement techniques (*see* Insertion of Arterial Line).

- Advantages
  - *Continuous*: it does not need repeated nurse measurements
  - *Accurate*: even when patients are profoundly hypotensive
  - *Other*: indications about myocardial contractility from the 'arterial swing' of the arterial trace can be evaluated (*see* Insertion of Arterial Line)
- Disadvantages
  - *Complications*: it is an invasive procedure in an artery under high pressure
  - *Skilled*: requires a degree of technical skill and full aseptic non-touch sterile technique
  - *Expensive*: it costs more than NIBP

Draw the blood pressure waveform

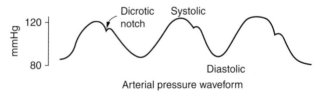

Figure 3.1

The dicrotic notch is a momentary rise in the arterial pressure trace following closure of the aortic valve.

How is the mean arterial pressure (MAP) calculated?

The area beneath the arterial pressure wave tracing represents the mean arterial pressure and is calculated

$$MAP = DP + 1/3 \, (SP - DP)$$

DP is the diastolic pressure and SP is the systolic pressure.

What information can be acquired from the shape of the arterial waveform?

In addition to measuring the blood pressure, the shape of the waveform gives further useful information

- *Myocardial contractility*: the rate of change of pressure by unit time, i.e. the slope of the arterial upstroke
- *Hypovolaemia*: this is suggested by a narrow waveform, a low dicrotic notch and a peak pressure, which varies with respiration if the patient is ventilated (or deep inspirations in the spontaneously breathing patient). This is the so-called 'arterial swing'

What is Allen's test and how is it performed?

Allen's test evaluates the competence of the collateral circulation of the hand. It is used to determine if the ulnar artery supply to the hand is able to cope in the face of an absent radial artery, e.g. when considering the use of the radial artery as a vascular conduit for bypass surgery, ABG analysis or arterial line insertion.

Blood flow is occluded by pressing on both the radial and ulnar fossae while the patient drains the hand of blood by repeatedly opening and closing the fist. The hand is then held open while ulnar flow is released. It is positive if the hand is still blanched after 15 seconds, suggesting the ulnar artery alone is not able to sufficiently supply the hand.

How does the arterial pressure at the radial artery compare to that at the aortic root and what accounts for this difference?

Both the pressure values and the waveform change at different levels of the circulation. In the radial artery the SP is ~10 mmHg higher and the DP ~10 mmHg lower than in the aortic root. Despite the pulse pressure (PP) being higher in the radial artery (PP = SP – DP), the MAP is ~5 mmHg lower than in the aortic root. These changes are due to differential wall stiffness throughout the arterial tree and its effect on pulse wave transmission in the vessel.

How does the arterial pressure waveform differ with diseases of the aortic valve?

- *Aortic stenosis*: anacrotic pulse, slow to rise and of low amplitude
- *Aortic incompetence*: water hammer pulse, rapid rise and decline, but attaining high amplitude
- *Mixed aortic valve disease*: pulsus bisferiens, a large amplitude pulse with a double peak, often felt as a double pulse at the brachial artery

What is pulsus alternans?

Pulsus alternans is a random variation in the amplitude of the arterial pressure tracing palpated as strong and weak beats during each cardiac cycle, e.g. during left ventricular failure, cardiomyopathy or aortic stenosis.

What is pulsus bisferiens?

Pulsus bisferiens is palpated as a double peak during the cardiac cycle. It classically exists in mixed aortic valve disease, e.g. aortic regurgitation and aortic stenosis.

What is pulsus paradoxus?

Pulsus paradoxus is a >10 mmHg reduction in arterial pressure caused by inspiration and may be seen in cardiac tamponade, e.g. a tight pericardial space leads to a reduction of left ventricular end-diastolic volume (LVEDV) and stroke volume, despite the usual increase in venous return during inspiration, which causes a <10 mmHg drop.

Blood products

What blood products exist?

The other major blood products are classified as

- Blood components
  - Red cells
  - Platelets
  - Fresh frozen plasma (FFP), including platelet concentrates
  - Cryoprecipitate
- Plasma derivatives
  - Human albumin solution (HAS)

- Coagulation factor concentrates
- Immunoglobulin (used in medical as opposed to surgical patients)

Blood components are prepared in blood transfusion centres and plasma derivatives are manufactured from pooled plasma from multiple donors in pooled fractionation centres. Both are covered by the Medicines Act.

What are the basic constituents and characteristics of a unit of packed red cells?

Red cells are used to restore the oxygen-carrying capacity and must be ABO compatible to the recipient

- *Volume*: 220–340 ml
- *Storage temperature*: 2–6°C
- *Shelf life*: 35 days from donation and the correct temperature
- *Haemoglobin content*: 40 g
- *Haematocrit*: 0.5–0.7

The most common additive solution is 100 ml *s*aline, *a*denine, *g*lucose and *m*annitol solution (SAG-M). This enables re-suspension of the packed red cells once the plasma has been removed and maintains cell integrity.

How are red cells treated to decrease disease transmission and allergic reactions?

- *Irradiation*: for patients at risk of transfusion-associated graft vs. host disease (TA-GvHD) (*see* Blood Transfusion) using γ-rays <14 days of donation (shelf life <14 days)

- *Washings*: plasma is removed and the cells re-suspended in 100 ml SAG-M if patients have recurrent allergic (or febrile) reactions, IgA deficiency and have anti-IgA deficient antibodies (shelf life <24 h)

What are the indications for transfusing a pack of red cells?
The indications include causes that decrease the oxygen-carrying capacity of the blood, e.g. hypovolaemic shock secondary to blood loss in cases of trauma, symptomatic anaemia.

What are the basic constituents and characteristics of a unit of platelets?
Platelets are used to treat bleeding secondary to platelet loss, consumption or platelet dysfunction. An adult therapeutic dose (ATD) is 240×10^9. Each donation produces 55×10^9, and platelets are produced in two ways

- Multiple blood donors
    - *Centrifuged*: four donations are pooled in the plasma of one of the donors. This reduces the risk of transfusion-related acute lung injury (TRALI) (*see* Blood Transfusion)
- Single blood donor
    - *Apheresis*: where donors may give multiple donations in a single session

It is preferable to provide >80% of donations through apheresis to reduce exposure to multiple donors, e.g. vCJD transmission.

Multiple donors

- *No. of donors per pack*: 4
- *Volume*: 300 ml
- *Storage temperature*: 20–24°C and agitation
- *Shelf life*: 5 days (7 days if bacterial screening)
- *Mean platelets*: 308 × 10^9 (range 165–500)

Single donors

- *No. of donors per pack*: 1
- *Volume*: around 200 ml
- *Storage temperature*: 20–24°C and agitation
- *Shelf life*: 5 days (7 days if bacterial screening)
- *Mean platelets*: 280 × 10^9 (range 165–510)

How are platelets treated to decrease disease transmission and allergic reactions?

- *Irradiation*: for patients at risk of TA-GvHD (*see* Blood Transfusion), but platelets retain their normal shelf life, unlike red cells
- *Washings*: plasma is removed and the cells re-suspended in 200 ml of platelet additive solution (PAS) if patients have recurrent allergic (or febrile) reactions (shelf life <24 h)
- *Human leucocyte antigen (HLA)-selected patients*: indicated for patients' refractory to treatment due to developing HLA antibodies following previous transfusions. Blood Services maintain a panel of HLA-typed platelet donors, e.g. but apheresis, and irradiation also occurs

- *Human platelet antigen (HPA)-selected patients*: HPA-1a/5b negative platelets are stored for use in neonatal alloimmune thrombocytopaenia (NAIT)

What are the indications for transfusing a pack of platelets?

The indications include any cause of thrombocytopaenia, e.g. $<50 \times 10^9$, disseminated intravascular coagulation (DIC) and post-cardiopulmonary bypass. This decreased platelet number and the cooling reduces platelet function. Aspirin is a common preoperative factor reducing platelet number.

What are the basic constituents and characteristics of a unit of plasma?

Plasma is only obtained from male donors to reduce the risk of TRALI. It is used to treat bleeding due to multiple clotting factor deficiencies. Two variants exists

- Single donor
  - *Fresh frozen plasma (FFP)*: its main components are cryoprecipitate and cryosupernatant containing all coagulation, von Willebrand's factor and some plasma proteins, e.g. fibrinogen
- Multiple donors
  - *Solvent detergent fresh frozen plasma (SD-FFP)*: e.g. Octoplas® pooled from ~1520 vCJD low-risk donors.

The dose of FFP is 10–15 ml/kg. It should not be used as a plasma volume expander due to carrying a significant risk of allergic reactions. It is no longer indicated in reversal of warfarin.

Single donors

- *No. of donors per pack*: 1
- *Volume*: around 275 ml
- *Storage temperature*: −25°C
- *Shelf life*: 36 months (24 h at 4°C days after thawing)
- *Mean Factor VIIIc*: 0.83 iU/ml

Multiple donors

- *No. of donors per pack*: 1520 max
- *Volume*: 200 ml
- *Storage temperature*: −18°C
- *Shelf life*: 4 years (transfuse immediately after thawing)
- *Mean Factor VIIIc*: 0.8 iU/ml
- *Mean fibrinogen*: 2.6 mg/ml

How is plasma treated to decrease disease transmission and allergic reactions?

- *Methylene blue*: e.g. SD-FFP inactivates bacteria-encapsulated viruses, e.g. HBV, HCV and HIV. It significantly reduces the incidence of allergic reactions and TRALI, but decreases concentrations of Factor VIIIc and fibrinogen 15–20%, and levels of Protein S are 30% lower.

What are the indications for transfusing a pack of platelets?

The indications include disseminated intravascular coagulation (DIC), inherited clotting factor deficiencies, e.g. Factor V Leiden deficiency, antithrombin deficiency, resistance to heparin, following massive blood transfusion, intraoperative and post-operative bleeding.

What are the basic constituents and characteristics of a pack of cryoprecipitate?

Cryoprecipitate is the supernatant obtained by thawing FFP at 4°C. It contains fibrinogen, von Willebrand's factor, Factor VIIIc and Factor XIII (fibrin-stabilising factor). Two variants exist

Single donors

- *No. of donors per pack*: 1
- *Volume*: around 40 ml
- *Storage temperature*: –25°C
- *Shelf life*: 36 months (transfuse immediately after thawing and do not refrigerate)
- *Mean Factor VIIIc*: 105 iU/pack
- *Mean fibrinogen*: 400 mg/pack

Multiple donors

- *No. of donors per pack*: 5
- *Volume*: 190 ml
- *Storage temperature*: –25°C
- *Shelf life*: 36 months (transfuse immediately after thawing and do not refrigerate)
- *Mean Factor VIIIc*: 464 iU/pack
- *Mean fibrinogen*: 1550 mg/pack

The dose is 1 U per 5–10 kg of body weight and raises plasma fibrinogen by ∼1 g/L.

What are the indications for transfusing a pack of cryoprecipitate?

The main indication is to replace fibrinogen if the plasma level <1.0 g/L. It is mainly used as a more concentrated source of fibrinogen than FFP. Hence a lower volume of infusion is required.

What is human albumin solution (HAS) and what types are available?

HAS contains no clotting factors or blood group antibodies, i.e. cross-matching is not required and two variants exist

- *Isotonic solutions (4.5%)*: requiring volumes of 50–500 ml, used to replace plasma loss caused by burns, pancreatitis, trauma and to replace fluid in plasma exchange
- *Hypertonic solutions (20%)*: this requires smaller volumes of 50–100 ml and can be used to initiate a diuresis in hypoalbuminaemic patients, e.g. hepatic cirrhosis (or nephrotic syndrome), reduction of ascites in portal hypertension. It contains less sodium so is called 'salt poor' albumin

What are the indications for using HAS?

The clinical uses are controversial as crystalloid or synthetic colloidal plasma substitutes are alternatives for use as plasma expanders in acute blood loss. It should not be used to correct low serum albumin levels in disease as side effects include severe hypersensitivity reactions.

What are coagulation factor concentrates and their use in surgical patients?

Coagulation factor concentrates contain individual clotting factors. The assortment of Factors II (prothrombin), VII, XI and X is called prothrombin complex concentrate (PCC). It has replaced FFP as the recommended treatment for the rapid reversal of warfarin overdose due to its superior efficacy, ease of administration and decreased risk of allergic reactions and fluid overload.

For which infections is donated blood screened?

The following tests are mandatory

- Hepatitis B (HBV): HBsAg
- Hepatitis C (HCV): anti-HCV and HCV NAT (nucleic acid testing)
- Human immunodeficiency virus (HIV): anti-HIV 1 and 2 and HIV NAT
- Human T-cell lymphocyte virus (HTLV): anti-HTLV 1 and 2
- Syphilis

In special circumstances, e.g. for use in the immunocompromised, cytomegalovirus (CMV) is screened. The above descriptions of blood products are based on information and guidelines from Joint United Kingdom (UK) Blood Transfusion and Tissue Transplantation Services Professional Advisory Committee (JPAC).

All blood donations are filtered to remove leucocytes (i.e. pre-storage leucodepletion) to leave $<1 \times 10^6$ leucocytes per pack), reducing the vCJD risk.

What is the management of PCC in warfarin overdose?

The management of warfarin overdose depends on the severity of the blood loss and the international normalised ratio (INR).

- No haemorrhage
  - *INR 4.5–6.0*: reduce the dose (or stop warfarin) and restart once INR <5
  - *INR 6–8*: stop warfarin and restart once INR <5
  - *INR >8*: if no bleeding or minor bleeding, stop warfarin. If risk factors exist, give 0.5–2.5 mg vitamin K orally (or as an infusion)
- Major haemorrhage
  - *INR >1.1*: conduct immediate ABCDE assessment and stop warfarin. Dual pharmacological treatment includes 5–10 mg vitamin K as an IV infusion in 5% dextrose and PCC, e.g. 25–50 iU/kg of Octaplex® (max dose 3000 U). Re-check INR 15–30 minutes after PCC and 4–6 hours after vitamin K administration. Only if PCC is unavailable can FFP be given (15 ml/kg)

In all cases of major haemorrhage contact the on-call haematologist to both administer PCC and discuss a plan to reintroduce anticoagulation once bleeding has stopped. A cause also needs to be searched.

Blood transfusion

What is the purpose of a blood transfusion?

To restore the circulating volume in order to improve tissue perfusion and to maintain an adequate blood oxygen-carrying capacity.

What is the expected increase in the haemoglobin concentration [Hb] following a transfusion of packed red cells?

A 4 ml/kg dose of packed cells raises the [Hb] by 1 g/dL.

How may the complications of blood transfusion be classified?

- Complications of massive transfusion
- Complications of repeated transfusion
- Infective complications
- Immune complications

Define massive transfusion and what are the potential problems?

A massive transfusion is defined as a transfusion equalling the patients' blood volume within 24 hours. The potential problems are

- *Volume overload*: which can lead to worsening pulmonary oedema in the susceptible
- *Thrombocytopaenia*: following storage there is a reduction in the functioning platelets, so that there is a dilutional thrombocytopaenia following a large transfusion
- *Coagulation factor deficiency*: leading to a coagulopathy, which may require blood products such as FFP for reversal
- *Poor tissue oxygenation*: due to reduction of 2,3-bisphosphoglycerate, which does not store well
- *Hypothermia*: due to cold-stored blood products being rapidly infused

- *Hypocalcaemia*: due to chelation by the citrate in the additive solution, which may compound the coagulation defect
- *Hyperkalaemia*: due to progressive potassium leakage from the stored red cells

These can also occur in repeated transfusions, in addition to the development of secondary haemochromatosis.

Which coagulation factors are most affected by storage?

The most labile of the coagulation factors are V and VIIIc. The reduction of Factor VIIIc may be offset by the metabolic response to stress, which stimulates Factor VIIIc production.

What infective complications may be seen following transfusion?

- Viruses, e.g. HBV, HCV and HIV
- Bacteria
  - Gram-negative, e.g. *Yersinia enterocolitica*, often implicated in red cell transfusions
  - Gram-positive, e.g. especially staphylococcal following contamination
- Syphilis
- Tropical disease, e.g. malaria, Chagas disease

What would make you suspect that a unit of blood has bacterial contamination?

- Presence of clots in the bag
- High degree of haemolysed red cells

Bacterial contamination reactions are rare, but often occur due to red cells stored at 2–6°C, which can be rapidly fatal. It can produce lethal septic shock depending on the species.

Which immune reactions may occur following transfusion?

Immune reactions can be classified as severe, less severe or delayed.

Severe life-threatening reactions

- *Acute haemolytic transfusion reactions*: e.g. ABO incompatibility, usually due to a clerical error. Transfusion of ABO-incompatible red cells react with the patient's anti-A or anti-B antibodies, resulting in rapid destruction of the transfused red cells (intravascular haemolysis) and release of inflammatory cytokines
- *Anaphylactic reactions*: this can include a mild urticaria to shock, or severe hypotension, bronchospasm, stridor from laryngeal oedema or life-threatening angio-oedema
- *Allergic reactions (IgA deficiency)*: this occurs in only a small minority of patients, and those most at risk have severe IgA deficiency (<0.07 g/L)
- *Transfusion-related acute lung injury (TRALI)*: this is classically caused by antibodies in donor blood reacting to neutrophils, monocytes or pulmonary endothelium. Inflammatory cells, sequestered in the lungs, cause non-cardiogenic pulmonary oedema
- *Transfusion-associated circulatory overload (TACO)*: is acute pulmonary oedema in <6 hours post-transfusion, and

features include acute respiratory distress, tachycardia,
hypertension and fluid overload

Less life-threatening reactions

- *Febrile non-haemolytic transfusion reaction (FNHTR)*:
  occurs within an hour of commencement as a reaction to
  leucocyte antigens in the donated blood. It is characterised
  by pyrexia, shivering, myalgia

Delayed reactions

- *Delayed haemolytic transfusion reaction (DHTR)*: occurs in
  under 24 hours, as the patient is immunised to foreign red
  cell antigens due to previous exposure, and can lead to
  jaundice and haemolysis days later
- *Post-transfusion purpuric reaction (PTP)*: occurs 5–12 days
  following transfusion due to reaction to human platelet
  antigen 1a (HPA-1a)
- *Tissue-associated graft vs. host disease (TA-GvHD)*: can occur
  7–14 days later and, although rare, is a uniformly fatal
  reaction. Immunocompetent donor lymphocytes mediate
  an immune reaction to recipient cells of a different HLA type

How is the risk of TA-GvHD reduced?

This is prevented by irradiation of the sample, and not simply
through the use of leucocyte-depleted blood.

**What are the signs and symptoms of an immediate
haemolytic transfusion reaction?**

- Pyrexia and rigors

- Headache
- Abdominal and loin pain
- Facial flushing
- Hypotension, progressing to acute kidney injury, disseminated intravascular coagulation (DIC) and acute lung injury

How is an immediate haemolytic transfusion reaction managed, and which investigations would you perform?

This requires immediate ABCDE assessment, ordering the relevant investigations and contacting the on-call haematologist for advice

- Stop the transfusion immediately
- Commence IV fluid resuscitation, ensuring that the urine output is greater than 30–40 ml/kg/h
- Repeat grouping on the pre- and post-transfusion recipient sample
- Repeat the cross-match
- Perform a direct antiglobulin (Coomb's test) on the recipient's post-transfusion sample
- Look for the presence of DIC, e.g. increased fibrin degradation products, coagulopathy
- Check for evidence of the response to intravascular haemolysis, e.g. hyperbilirubinaemia, reduced circulating haptoglobins, haemoglobinaemia and haemoglobinuria
- Send samples for blood culture in case this was, in fact, a septic episode in response to contaminated blood

What is a direct Coomb's test?

Coomb's test, also known as a direct antiglobulin test (dAg), is used for the detection of antibody or complement on the surface of red cells that have developed *in vivo*. The indirect Coomb's test detects red cells binding that have developed *in vitro*. The direct test can be used in the detecting of cases of

- Haemolytic transfusion reactions
- Haemolytic disease of the newborn
- Autoimmune haemolytic anaemia

What are the problems associated with platelet transfusion?

- *Risk of infection*: as for a transfusion of packed red cells
- *Risk of sensitisation*: Rhesus (Rh) negative females under the age of 45 should receive Rh-D negative platelets
- *Alloimmunisation*: this is due to development of antibodies to HLA class I antigens. It can lead to a febrile transfusion reaction and refractoriness to therapy, when the platelet count rises less than expected following transfusion

ECG: basic concepts

What are the anatomic locations of the sinoatrial (SA) and atrioventricular (AV) nodes?

The SA node is an elliptical area found at the junction of the superior vena cava and the right atrium. The AV node is found in the triangular area of the right atrial wall just above the septal cusp of the tricuspid valve.

Where on the body are the ECG leads placed?

The locations of the electrodes are

- Bipolar (limb) leads
  - Red: right wrist
  - Yellow: left wrist
  - Black: right ankle
  - Green: left ankle
- Unipolar (chest) leads
  - V1: 4th intercostal space, right of the sternum
  - V2: 4th intercostal space, left of the sternum
  - V3: midway between V2 and V4
  - V4: normal apex, left 5th intercostal space, mid-clavicular line
  - V5: anterior axillary line at the level of V4
  - V6: mid-axillary line at the level of V4

Draw a typical ECG waveform, and label the various reflections

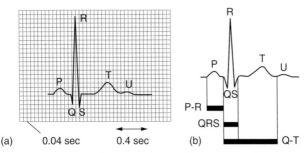

Figure 3.2 (a) Normal ECG complexes. (b) P-R, QRS and QT segments. Reproduced with permission from *Cardiology*, 6th edn. Edited by Julian and Cowan (1992), p. 14. Published by Baillière Tindall, ISBN 0702016446.

When do the heart sounds occur in relation to the electrical cycle of the heart?

The 1st heart sound, following closure of the AV valves, is heard at the end of the R-wave on the ECG. The 2nd heart sound, following closure of the VA valves, is heard at the end of the T-wave on the ECG.

What is the origin of the P-wave?

The P-wave is caused by atrial depolarisation. NB. It is not due to activity at the SA node.

Define the PR interval. What does it represent and what is the normal range?

The PR interval is measured from the beginning of the P-wave to the beginning of the QRS complex. It corresponds to the time taken for the impulse to travel from the SA node to the ventricle. The normal range is 0.12–0.20 seconds (3–5 small squares). A prolonged PR interval indicates heart block.

What does the QRS interval represent and what is the upper limit of its duration?

The QRS complex represents ventricular muscle depolarisation and the upper limit is 0.12 seconds. A widened QRS >0.12 seconds can be caused by conduction delays, e.g. bundle branch block.

Define the QT interval

The QT interval is from the start of the QRS complex to the end of the T-wave. It represents the time from the onset of ventricular depolarisation to full repolarisation. Its duration is heart-rate dependent.

What is the QTc interval and how is it calculated?

The QTc interval is the QT interval that has been corrected for variations in the heart rate. It represents the QT interval standardised to a heart rate of 60 bpm, permitting comparisons between individuals. Using Bazett's formula: $QTc = QT/\sqrt{(RR)}$. At a heart rate of 60 bpm the $QTc = QT$ and has a normal range of 0.35–0.43 seconds.

What does the T-wave represent and why is its deflection in the same direction as the QRS complex?

The T-wave represents ventricular myocardial repolarisation. Since it represents repolarisation, one would expect the deflection to be negative. However, repolarisation occurs from the epicardium to endocardium, which is in the opposite direction. This causes the deflection to be in the same direction as for depolarisation.

Have you heard of J- and U-waves? Where in the electrical cycle may they appear and under what circumstances may they be seen?

- *J-wave*: the J-point of the normal ECG is found at the junction of the S-wave and the ST segment. A J-wave is an upward deflection found at this point, and may be seen in hypothermia

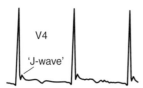

Figure 3.3 Reproduced with permission from the *Oxford Handbook of Clinical Medicine*, 8th edn. Edited by Longmore et al. (2010). Published by Oxford University Press, ISBN 9780199232178.

- *U-wave*: this is a low voltage wave found after the T-wave of some normal individuals, but can become more prominent in cases of hypokalaemia

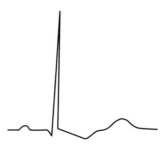

Figure 3.4

ECG: complex concepts

Give some causes of sinus tachycardia (HR >100 bpm)

- Exercise
- Pain (and anxiety)
- Pyrexia, e.g. T° >38°C
- Shock (of any cause)
- Hyperthyroidism

- Anaemia
- Drugs
  - Catecholamines, e.g. adrenaline, noradrenaline, dopamine
  - Atropine
  - Aminophylline

Give some causes of sinus bradycardia (HR <60 bpm)
- Athletic heart syndrome
- Vasovagal
- Hypothermia
- Hypothyroidism
- Raised intracranial pressure (as part of the Cushing reflex)
- Jaundice
- Drugs
  - β-blockers
  - Digoxin
  - Amiodarone

What kinds of tachyarrhythmias do you know?
- Broad complex
  - *Regularly broad complex tachycardia*: this is most likely due to ventricular tachycardia (VT) or a supraventricular tachycardia (SVT) in bundle branch block
  - *Irregularly broad complex tachycardia*: the most likely cause is atrial fibrillation (AF) in bundle branch block. Other causes include AF in ventricular pre-excitation, e.g. Wolff–Parkinson–White (WPW) syndrome, polymorphic VT

- Narrow complex
  - *Regular narrow complex tachycardia*: this includes the non-pathological sinus tachycardia, and paroxysmal SVT, e.g. atrioventricular re-entry tachycardia (AVRT) such as WFW syndrome and atrial flutter in *regular* AV conduction block, e.g. 2:1
  - *Irregularly narrow complex tachycardia*: the most common cause of this particular SVT is AF. Atrial flutter in *variable* AV conduction block, e.g. 2:1, 3:1 or 4:1, may also occur

What are the characteristic features of an SVT?
- Heart rate >150–220 bpm
- QRS complex duration <0.12 s
- P-waves may be abnormal shape or absent altogether

What are the characteristic features of atrial flutter?
- Atrial rate >250–350 bpm
- QRS complexes are of normal morphology
- P-waves are '*sawtooth*' shaped

How are attacks of tachyarrhythmias managed?
They are managed according to the Advanced Life Support (ALS) protocol and depends on the presence (or absence) of adverse features, e.g. shock, syncope, myocardial ischaemia and heart failure, and if the rhythm is broad or narrow complex. All cases require immediate ABCDE assessment, continuous ECG, blood pressure and SaO_2 monitoring and a 12-lead ECG once the episode has stopped.

If no adverse features exist

- Broad complex
  - *Regularly broad complex tachycardia*: e.g. VT give 300 mg of amiodarone IV in a large vein over 20–60 minutes then 900 mg over 24 hours
  - *Irregularly broad complex tachycardia*: seek expert help urgently
- Narrow complex
  - *Regularly narrow complex tachycardia*: e.g. paroxysmal SVT, use carotid sinus massage. If it persists give 6 mg of adenosine IV stat in a large vein. If no response give 12 mg of adenosine (can be repeated once)
  - *Irregularly narrow complex tachycardia*: e.g. AF, give 50 mg of metoprolol (1st line) or 500 μg (micrograms) digoxin (2nd line), which is a loading dose. Consider anticoagulation

If adverse features exist (and a pulse is present)

- Synchronised DC shock (repeated three times)
- Give 300 mg of amiodarone in a large vein over 10–20 minutes and repeat the shock, followed by 900 mg over 24 hours

If the patient has recurrent cases of a stable tachyarrhythmia, cardiac catheterisation can ablate the focus.

How are attacks of bradyarrhythmias managed?
They are managed according to the Advanced Life Support (ALS) protocol and depends on the presence (or absence) of

adverse features, e.g. shock, syncope, myocardial ischaemia and heart failure, and if the rhythm is broad or narrow complex. All cases require immediate ABCDE assessment, continuous ECG, blood pressure and SaO_2 monitoring and a 12-lead ECG once the episode has stopped.

If no adverse features exist

- Risk of asystole, e.g. recent asystole, complete heart block, ventricular pause >3 seconds
  - *Yes*: interim measures (*see* below)
  - *No*: observe

If adverse features exist (and a pulse is present)

- Give 500 µg (micrograms) atropine and a response does exist
  - *Yes*: assess for risk of asystole (*as* above)
  - *No*: conduct interim measures which include repeated doses of 500 µg (micrograms) of atropine to a max dose of 3 mg, 5 µg (micrograms)/min of isoprenaline, 2–10 µg (micrograms)/min of adrenaline. Seek expert help as transcutaneous, or transvenous, pacing may be required. Complete heart block is managed using a permanent pacemaker

Draw basic rhythm strips of hearts exhibiting 1st degree, 2nd degree and complete (3rd degree) AV block, identifying the defining morphology

First degree heart block: a prolonged PR interval that is fixed in duration.

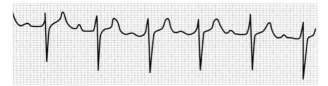

Figure 3.5 First degree heart block.
Reproduced with permission from the *Oxford Handbook of Clinical Medicine*, 8th edn. Edited by Longmore et al. (2010). Published by Oxford University Press, ISBN 9780199232178.

- Prolonged PR interval
- Constant in timing
- Always followed by a QRS complex

Second degree heart block: Mobitz Type I (Wenckebach phenomenon): the PR interval becomes progressively more prolonged, until one of the P-waves is not followed by a QRS complex. After this, the cycle repeats itself.

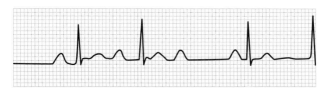

Figure 3.6 Second degree heart block (Mobitz Type I).
Reproduced with permission from the *Oxford Handbook of Clinical Medicine*, 8th edn. Edited by Longmore et al. (2010). Published by Oxford University Press, ISBN 9780199232178.

- Progressive lengthening of the PR interval
- Until a P-wave fails to be conducted

Second degree heart block: Mobitz Type II: some of the P-waves are not followed by a QRS, and this is consistent between beats, e.g. 2:1, 3:1, etc.

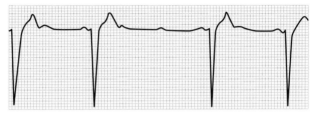

Figure 3.7 Second degree heart block (Mobitz Type II). Reproduced with permission from the *Oxford Handbook of Clinical Medicine*, 8th edn. Edited by Longmore et al. (2010). Published by Oxford University Press, ISBN 9780199232178.

- PR intervals remain unchanged
- Prior to an occasional P-wave that does not conduct

Third degree heart block: complete: there is no recognisable relationship between the P-waves and the onset of the QRS complexes.

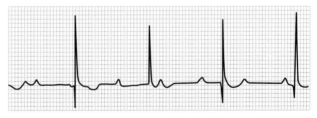

Figure 3.8 Third degree heart block (complete). Reproduced with permission from the *Oxford Handbook of Clinical Medicine*, 8th edn. Edited by Longmore et al. (2010). Published by Oxford University Press, ISBN 9780199232178.

- P-waves bear no relationship to the QRS complex
- Therefore, atria and ventricles function independently

Fluid therapy

How do you assess the state of hydration?

There are multiple ways to assess hydration, but in case of clinical concern, immediate ABCDE assessment is required. In fluid assessment

Clinical examination of the patient

- Underfilled
  - Cool peripheries
  - ↓Capillary refill time (>2 s)
  - Tachycardia
  - ↓Skin turgor
  - Hypotension, e.g. a postural drop
  - Dry mouth
  - Sunken eyes
  - ↓Urine output (<30 ml/min/kg)
- Overfilled
  - ↑JVP
  - Tachypnoea
  - Bibasal fine end-inspiratory crepitations, e.g. in pulmonary oedema
  - Pitting oedema of the sacrum, ankles, legs and abdomen

Inspection of bedside scores, charts and lines

- Early Warning Score (EWS) (or SEWS in Scotland)

- Tachycardia and if a persistent HR >100 bpm has existed
- Hypotension and the presence of a gradual drop in systolic BP <90 mmHg
- Fluid balance chart
  - Oral intake and if fluid has been enteral or parenteral
  - Urinary catheter to assess urinary volume and concentration
  - Surgical drains to look for potential blood losses post-operatively
- Central venous pressure (CVP)
  - Its measurement (0–10 mmHg) and response to a fluid challenge. If there is under filling, the CVP will not increase following a challenge

What are the main fluid compartments of the body and what are their volumes?

The fluid compartments are

- *Intracellular compartment*: 28 L
- *Extracellular compartment*: 14 L composed of 3 L plasma, 10 L interstitium and 1 L transcellular fluid

The total body water is 42 L and makes up ∼60% of the body weight of a 70 kg male and 55–60% of a female. The basal requirements for an adult are 30–40 ml/kg/day.

What is the purpose of fluid therapy?

An average person requires ∼2500 ml of fluid in 24 hours and losses include 1500 ml as urine, 200 ml as stool and 800 ml as insensible losses, e.g. respiration, perspiration (even inspiration). This requirement is usually obtained through 1000 ml from food and 1500 ml from drink. Therefore, the purpose of fluid therapy is to

- Satisfy basal requirements of water and electrolytes (*see* Chapter 5, Renal)
- Replace lost fluid and electrolytes
- Support arterial pressure in cases of shock by increasing the plasma volume and improving tissue perfusion
- Increase the oxygen-carrying capacity of the blood, e.g. if red cells are infused

By which routes may fluids be administered?

The main routes are dictated by the clinical context and the functional status of the patient

- Enteral
  - Mouth
- Parenteral
  - Intravenous (IV), but carries a risk of infection, e.g. femoral > jugular > ante-cubital
  - Subcutaneous (SC), particularly if IV access is difficult, e.g. in palliation
  - Intraosseous (IO) using a metal cannula into the medullary cavity of the tibia, e.g. in trauma, if IV access is difficult to obtain due to peripheral circulatory shutdown

What types of fluids are available?

Fluids may be given as

- *Colloids*: these may be naturally occurring or synthetic and confine themselves to the plasma, exerting an osmotic pressure (unless there is injury to capillary integrity resulting in leakage into the interstitium)
- *Crystalloid*: these solutions are able to more easily pass between compartments. In the case of 5% dextrose, once it has been metabolised, the remaining water distributes itself in the total body water

Would you use crystalloids or colloids in the emergency setting?

This is a controversial issue. Both are able to provide plasma volume expansion in the support of the arterial pressure during blood loss. Crystalloids have no oxygen-carrying capacity, unlike red cells (a colloid). This is likely to be required in cases of severe blood loss, which diminishes tissue oxygenation. Also, because of the volume of distribution of crystalloid, more of it is required than colloid to provide a comparable increase in the plasma volume.

What types of crystalloid are available and what are the basic characteristics of each?

The crystalloids available are

- *Saline (0.9%)*: has 150 mmol/L each of sodium and chloride. It is isotonic and has an osmolality of 300 mOsm/L and a pH of 5. It rapidly equilibrates in vascular spaces and is suitable for resuscitation. It is cheap but effective

- *Hartmann's (compound sodium lactate)*: contains 131 mmol/L sodium, 5 mmol/L potassium, 111 mmol/L chloride, 29 mmol/L bicarbonate (lactate metabolised) and 2 mmol/L calcium. It has an osmolality of 280 mOsm/L and a pH of 6.5 and is considered more physiological
- *Dextrose (5%)*: is isotonic and contains 50 g/L glucose, which is rapidly metabolised by the liver and equilibrates throughout all fluid compartments. It is useless for resuscitation but each litre provides ~10% daily energy requirements. It has a pH of 4

What are the precautions with using crystalloids?

- *Metabolic acidosis*: this is due to hyperchloraemia resulting from excessive saline use and the associated *chloride shift*, particularly in renal insufficiency
- *Hyperkalaemia*: can occur from prolonged use of Hartmann's solutions in patients predisposed to hyperkalaemia, e.g. renal failure
- *Hypernatraemia*: if hypertonic saline, e.g. 10% solution is used intraoperatively or in trauma. It requires judicious use and comes in 1.8%, 3%, 5% and 7.5% preparations
- *Oedema*: occurs if excess dextrose solution is used, as it does not preferentially remain in the intravascular space, e.g. contraindicated in cerebral oedema

What types of colloid are available and what are the basic characteristics of each?

The colloids available are

- *Human albumin solution (4.5% or 20%)*: obtained by fractionation of plasma and provides plasma expansion. Its plasma $t_{1/2}$ 1.6 hours ($\sim$20 days in the body). The 4.5% preparation is isotonic and can produce a five times increase of its own volume in 30 minutes (pH 7.4)
- *Dextrans (40 or 70 depending on the molecular weight)*: artificial colloids composed of branched polysaccharides. It can be used as a volume expander and the dose is <20 ml/kg/day, but mostly used as an antiaggregant in microvascular surgery. Its plasma $t_{1/2}$ $\sim$12 hours (pH 5)
- *Gelatins*: formed from the hydrolysis of bovine collagen. Its plasma $t_{1/2}$ $\sim$2–4 hours being rapidly excreted by the kidneys but have a long shelf life (<3 years). There are three main types
  - Succinylated gelatins, e.g. Gelofusin
  - Urea cross-linked gelatins, e.g. Haemaccel
  - Oxypolygelatins
- *Starches*: include 6% hetastarch ($t_{1/2}$ 5 days) or pentastarch ($t_{1/2}$ 24 h) consisting of glucose molecule chains. They can be useful in cases of capillary leakage when smaller colloids may worsen interstitial oedema. The dose of hetastarch is limited to 1500 ml/day due to the risk of coagulopathy

What are the precautions with using colloids?
- *Potential risk of disease transmission*: in blood and blood products, e.g. human albumin solution (HAS)
- *Coagulopathy*: Dextran 70, gelatins and high molecular weight starches interfere with platelet adhesion and von Willebrand's factor, decrease Factor VIIIc and Factor V levels

- *Interaction with blood transfusion*: the calcium content of Haemaccel can cause blood to clot if infused into the same cannula
- *Immunological reactions*: other than blood, Dextran 70 and gelatins may cause pruritis or anaphylaxis
- *Volume overload*: there is a risk of worsening oedema if loss of capillary integrity causes the colloid to leak into the interstitial compartment

Jugular venous pulse (JVP)

Which of the jugular veins is used for examination of the JVP and why?

The internal jugular vein and its lack of valves, unlike in the external jugular, provides a single column of blood that is directly affected by events in the right heart and thoracic cavity.

What information may be obtained from an examination of the JVP?

The JVP provides a clinical measurement of the central venous pressure (CVP) of 0–10 mmHg. This equates to the right atrial pressure and provides information on circulatory volume and right ventricular function. Observing the waveform of the JVP may give information about the patient's heart rhythm and right heart function.

How may it be distinguished from the carotid pulse?

- There are two ('*a*' and '*v*') venous pulsations to each carotid pulse

- The venous pulse is obliterated by light pressure at the root of the neck
- The height of the JVP varies with the respiratory cycle
- Abdominal compression causes a momentary rise in the JVP (abdominal reflex)

Draw the normal JVP waveform explaining how the differing wave deflections come about

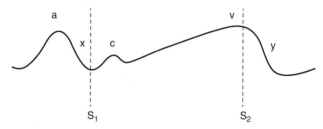

Figure 3.9 The jugular venous pulse waveform in relation to the first (S_1) and second (S_2) heart sounds.

What do the individual deflections represent?

- *a* wave is due to atrial contraction
- *x* descent is due to a fall in atrial pressure during ventricular systole
- *c* wave is produced by the bulging of the tricuspid valve into the atrium at the start of ventricular systole
- *v* wave occurs as a result of venous return to the atrium, i.e. atrial filling against a closed tricuspid valve
- *y* descent occurs at the opening of the tricuspid valve

What are the causes of an elevated JVP?

Some of the causes include

- Obstruction of flow into the right atrium, e.g. SVC obstruction due to a lung tumour, mediastinal mass or large goitre. There is also loss of the waveform
- Disease at the level of right AV function, e.g. tricuspid valvular stenosis, incompetence or a right atrial myxoma (rare)
- Compressed right ventricle, e.g. cardiac tamponade or constrictive pericarditis

How does the waveform differ in cases of atrial fibrillation, complete heart block, tricuspid stenosis and incompetence?

- *Atrial fibrillation*: absent '*a*' wave producing an irregularly irregular pulse
- *Complete heart block*: cannon '*a*' waves due to discordant atrial and ventricular contractions can result in the atrium contracting against a closed tricuspid valve. This transmits a large wave to the internal jugular
- *Tricuspid stenosis*: large '*a*' waves due to obstruction at the AV level and slow '*y*' descent due to slow atrial emptying
- *Tricuspid incompetence*: large '*v*' waves due to surging of right ventricular blood into the atrium through an incompetent valve during ventricular systole

Why does the height of the JVP vary with the respiratory cycle?

In inspiration the intrathoracic pressure falls (becomes more negative), increasing venous return to the heart. The JVP falls as the column of blood flows into the heart. During expiration the rise in the intrathoracic pressure reduces this venous return, causing an elevation in the JVP.

What is Kussmaul's sign?

Kussmaul's sign is a paradoxical rise in the JVP on inspiration. It occurs in situations where the right atrium cannot accommodate the increase in its venous return caused by a fall in the intrathoracic pressure on inspiration, e.g. in right heart failure and constrictive pericarditis.

Complex concepts

Aortic dissection

How are aortic dissections classified?

Aortic dissections may be classified according to the Stanford or DeBakey systems

- Standford
  - *Type A*: dissection involves the ascending aorta, and can extend into the aortic arch and descending aorta
  - *Type B*: involves the descending aorta only
- DeBakey
  - *Type I*: involves the ascending aorta, arch and descending aorta
  - *Type II*: confined to the ascending aorta
  - *Type III*: confined to the descending aorta, beyond the origin of the subclavian artery and two subtypes exist; IIIa extends down to the diaphragm and IIIb extends beyond it

The Stanford system is more clinically useful as it delineates two distinct groups for management: Type A dissections require surgery whereas Type B dissections are managed conservatively, e.g. medical treatment.

What are the pathological hallmarks of dissections?

The recognised findings on microscopy are

- *Myxoid degeneration*: loss of elastic fibres and replacement of the musculo-elastic tissue with a proteoglycan rich matrix
- *Cystic medial necrosis (medial wall degeneration)*: may be associated with injury or occlusion of the vasa vasorum

Dissections can result from an intimal transverse tear along the greater curvature of the aorta (∼10 cm from the valve) and propagation of blood into the media (inner two-thirds and the outer one-third), or from intramural haemorrhage and haematoma formation in the media followed by intimal perforation. Tears occur in aortic regions subjected to great stress and pressure fluctuations, e.g. in hypertension and aortic dilation.

Which conditions predispose to aortic dissection?

The predisposing risk factors are

Non-modifiable

- Genetic
  - *Age*: >50 years
  - *Sex*: male preponderance
  - *Marfan's syndrome*: there is defective cross-linking of collagen

- *Ehlers–Danlos syndrome*: defective pro-collagen formation
- *Loeys–Dietz syndrome*: autosomal dominant mutation affecting the TGF-β receptor
- *Pseudoxanthoma elasticum*: fragmentation of elastic fibres in the media

Modifiable

- Congenital
  - *Bicuspid aortic valve*: the cause is unknown
- Lifestyle
  - *Hypertension*: leading to increased shearing forces across the intima
  - *Pregnancy*: associated with microscopic changes in the media
  - *Traumatic*: deceleration injuries to the aorta
  - *Pharmacological*: cocaine use
- Iatrogenic
  - *Interventions*: cardiac catheterisation, aortic cannulation at cardiac surgery, aortic valve replacement

What are the effects of dissection?
Dissection can lead to a number of outcomes depending on differential involvement of the arterial tree

- Abdominal aorta
  - *Propagation*: leading to gut ischaemia if the mesenteric vessels are involved, or renal failure if the renal vessels are involved

- Intercostal (and lumbar) vessels
  - *Occlusion*: causing spinal cord ischaemia due to loss of the supply from the arteria radicularis magna
- Carotid vessels
  - *Propagation*: leading to ischaemic stroke
- Cardiac
  - *Involvement*: of coronary ostia and coronary arteries leads to angina and myocardial infarction, and of the aortic valve ring produces acute aortic regurgitation
  - *Rupture*: of the dissection into the pericardium causes cardiac tamponade, and of the pleura produces a haemothorax
- Others
  - *Compression*: of surrounding structures, such as the trachea, oesophagus or superior vena cava

The dissection may re-enter the lumen through another intimal tear, producing a double-barrelled aorta, and blood may re-enter the true lumen at any point. This makes it a communicating dissection.

What may the physical examination show?
Some findings on physical examination

- Signs
  - *Symptomatic pain*: Type A produces severe chest pain, whilst Type B produces back and abdominal pain
  - *Cardiogenic (or hypovolaemic) shock*: indicating significant loss of circulating blood volume, e.g. low systolic BP, tachycardia

- *Cardiac tamponade*: revealing rupture into the pericardium, e.g. muffled heart sounds, increased JVP, reduced arterial pressure and pulsus paradoxus
- *Neurological dysfunction*: indicating stroke or spinal cord involvement

Asymmetrical pulses and blood pressures may be recorded in the arms, due to dissection in the aortic arch, and a new diastolic murmur of aortic regurgitation auscultated. The patient can be in a lot of pain and distress.

Which investigations may be employed in making the diagnosis?

The purpose of ordering the investigations is to enable

- *Correct diagnosis*: from the list of differentials
- *Assessment*: of the dissection to help plan management
- *Discovery*: of the presence of complications, e.g. myocardial infarction and the presence of other co-morbidities that can complicate management

There are a number of investigations that help in establishing the diagnosis and assessing the severity

- *ECG*: establishes the presence of myocardial infarction and excludes cardiac differential diagnoses
- *CXR*: abnormal in 80% of cases and may show a widened mediastinum, displacement of the aortic knuckle, depression of the left main bronchus or a haemothorax
- *Cardiac angiography*: the gold standard that allows visualisation of ventricular and valve function, and permits

assessment of coronary anatomy. However, it is invasive and the contrast dye may worsen renal dysfunction in an otherwise critically ill patient

- *CT/MRI scanning*: has a sensitivity and specificity of >85% and >90% respectively. It permits spiral CT imaging but does not provide information on cardiac function
- *Transoesophageal echocardiography (TEE)*: it has a sensitivity and specificity of >95%. It has the advantage that it can be used at the bedside, and can assess cardiac function and valve involvement.

How is aortic dissection managed?

All cases require immediate ABCDE assessment and also

- *Fluid resuscitation*: to maintain the cardiac index and renal function, e.g. a urine output of 30–40 ml/h must be maintained. Fluid is given through a wide bore cannulae, e.g. 14-G (orange)
- *Cross-matching*: bloods should be taken to get a baseline Hb level, renal function and a 10 U cross-match for transfusion
- *Monitoring of filling pressures*: a central line should be inserted to assess the CVP and response to fluid resuscitation
- *Monitoring and control of arterial pressures*: an arterial line should be inserted to acquire beat to beat blood pressure recordings. The velocity of the ejection fraction and arterial pressure (<130 mmHg) should be controlled using esmolol, i.e. β-blockade, and labetalol, i.e. α- and β-blockade. The disadvantage of sodium nitroprusside is that it causes a

reflex tachycardia and increases the ejection velocity. This
increases the shearing forces on the intima propagating the
dissection

- *Escalation in care*: the patient should be transferred to a
  cardiology and cardiothoracic unit and if the GCS <8, in
  conjunction to profound haemodynamic instability,
  intubation and ventilation are required
- *Surgery (Type A)*: involves replacement of the diseased
  segment of aorta with a prosthetic graft. Aortic root
  involvement requires valve replacement (or re-suspension)
  and re-implantation of the coronary arteries. If the arch is
  involved, deep hypothermic circulatory arrest is required
  during repair to preserve cerebral function
- *Stenting (Type B)*: surgery is not indicated in Type B
  dissection, except if there is persistent intractable pain,
  aneurysmal expansion, peripheral complications and
  rupture

For Type A dissections, the death rate is 1–2%/hour and the
surgical mortality 10–15%. For Type B dissections, the surgical
mortality is slightly higher.

Cardiogenic shock

What is the definition of cardiogenic shock?

Cardiogenic shock is inadequate tissue perfusion from
myocardial dysfunction, e.g. heart failure, with cardiac index
(CI) <2.2 L/min/m^2, pulmonary artery capillary wedge
pressure (PACWP) >18 mmHg and the systolic BP <90 mmHg.

Hypoxia persists despite adequate intravascular volume replacement. It occurs in 5–8% of patients following an ST-segment elevated myocardial infarction (STEMI) and is the most common cause of death.

What are the complications of a STEMI?

- Shock, e.g. cardiogenic
- Arrhythmias, e.g. tachyarrhythmias, bradyarrythmias and heart block
- Mechanical
  - *Ventricular septal defect (VSD)*: resulting in acute right ventricular overload and pulmonary oedema
  - *Free wall rupture*: resulting in cardiac tamponade
  - *Papillary muscle rupture*: presenting as acute mitral or tricuspid regurgitation
  - *Left ventricular aneurysm*: and mural thrombus as a late presentation producing progressive cardiac failure, or systemic embolism leading to stroke, acute limb and mesenteric ischaemia resulting in bowel infarction
  - *Chronic heart failure*: due to long-term deterioration in ventricular function as part of the ongoing ischaemic process
- Immunological
  - *Pericarditis (Dressler's syndrome)*: occurring several weeks after infarction with chest pain and pyrexia

What are the risk factors and main causes of cardiogenic shock?

The main cause is a myocardial infarction (MI), but risk factors and causes include

Risk factors

- Genetic
  - *Age*: >55 years
- Cardiac
  - *Ischaemic heart disease (IHD)*: due to angina, previous MIs, multi-vessel coronary artery disease, pre-existing heart failure, left bundle branch block (LBBB) and hypertension
- Endocrine
  - *Diabetes mellitus*: due to the acceleration is atherosclerotic disease, renal failure and subsequent hypertension development, and the silent MIs that go undiagnosed
- Infection
  - *Myocarditis*: this can lead to systolic dysfunction. Also, infective endocarditis can produce valve rupture and acute incompetence

Causes

- Cardiac (primary)
  - *Anterior MI*: a large infarction produces abnormal ventricular wall motion and systolic dysfunction. Wall rupture produces cardiac tamponade
  - *Acute arrhythmias*: tachyarrhythmias can lead to shortened diastolic filling time and reduce cardiac output
- Non-cardiac (secondary)
  - *Obstruction to cardiac output*: this includes pulmonary emboli, tension pneumothorax and aortic dissection. Myocardial contusions can result
- Iatrogenic

- *Post-cardiac surgery and prolonged cardiopulmonary bypass*: this can lead to myocardial '*stunning*', which is a temporary reduction in the cardiac output despite restoration of myocardial perfusion

What are the clinical features of cardiogenic shock and how may it be distinguished from other causes of shock?

The clinical features demonstrate a shocked patient and include

- Reduced CI (<2.2 L/min/m^2)
  - Cool peripheries
  - ↓Capillary refill time (>2 s)
  - ↓Urine output (<30 ml/min/kg)
  - ↓Consciousness, e.g. GCS <8 from poor cerebral perfusion
- Elevated CVP (>10 mmHg)
  - Volume overload, e.g. pulmonary oedema
  - ↑JVP due to decreased cardiac output, e.g. cardiac tamponade
  - Hepatomegaly from hepatic congestion
- Reduced MAP (<50 mmHg)
  - ↓Systolic BP <90 mmHg

On auscultation a gallop rhythm of a 3rd heart sound exists and a 4th heart sound may be heard. A bruit may reveal the underlying cause, e.g. VSD or mitral regurgitation. Clinically, it may be difficult to distinguish from shock due to cardiac tamponade or pulmonary embolism, but its dominant feature is acute pulmonary oedema. This contrasts septic shock as cardiac output is increased; bounding pulses and warm peripheries exist, followed by a systolic BP drop, and the JVP not being elevated.

What is the pathophysiology of decompensating cardiogenic shock?

The pathophysiological basis lies in the Frank–Starling curve

- *Right shift*: reflecting a higher end-diastolic pressure and volume to achieve an equivalent stroke volume. The sympathetic compensatory increase in the heart rate and contractility leads to increased myocardial O_2 demand (NB. progressive lactic acidosis suppresses myocardial contractility)

This may be summarised by the following diagram

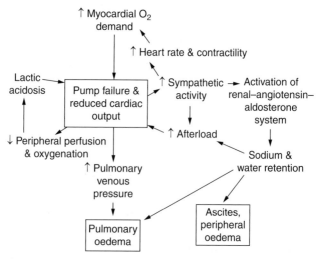

Figure 3.10

Which investigations are useful for cardiogenic shock?
All cases require immediate ABCDE assessment, continuous
ECG, blood pressure and SaO_2 monitoring. The following
investigations are useful in establishing the diagnosis and
severity

- *ECG*: for the presence of infarction or arrhythmia
- *CXR*: to assess for presence of hilar (bat's wing) and
  interstitial shadowing in pulmonary oedema, a widened
  mediastinum in cardiac tamponade or a dilated ventricle,
  prominent upper lobe vascular markings in venous
  congestion and left atrial enlargement due to a prominent
  left heart border
- *Transthoracic and transoesophageal echocardiography (TTE
  and TOE [TEE])*: may be performed at the bedside and
  demonstrate abnormal ventricular wall motion
- *CT*: can be used if a high degree of clinical suspicion
  suggests an acute aortic dissection, or a pulmonary embolus
- *Catheterisation*: of the pulmonary artery using a Swan–Ganz
  catheter to measure the PACWP and cardiac output. The
  insertion of central and arterial lines and urinary
  catheterisation enables fluid resuscitation, balance and
  blood pressure to be monitored

If the cause is a suspected acute MI, then transfer to a coronary
care unit (CCU) for percutaneous coronary intervention (PCI).
If this is not available, then thrombolysis is indicated. The
arterial pressure can be supported using pharmacological and
mechanical methods (*see* Chapter 6, Circulatory Support:
Inotropic Agents).

What information can be obtained from TTE and TOE (TEE)?

They provide the following information

- *Structural (static changes)*: such as the presence of valve lesions of a VSD
- *Functional (dynamic changes)*: colour-flow quantifies flow across a valve or septal defect, the calculation of pressure differences, ventricular contractility and function from end-systolic and end-diastolic measurements. TOE (TEE) provides a better picture of the left atrium and valve function

What are the findings from the pulmonary artery catheter in cardiogenic shock?

- ↑CVP
- CI <2.2 L/min/m^2
- PACWP >18 mmHg
- ↓Mixed venous congestion saturation

Coagulation defects

What are the basic components of normal haemostatic function?

Normal haemostatic function depends on the normal interplay of a number of components

- Normal vascular endothelium function and tissue integrity
- Normal platelet number and function
- Normal coagulation factor amount and function

- Presence of various essential agents, e.g. vitamin K and calcium
- Balanced relationship between the fibrinolytic pathway and the clotting cascade

What do platelets do and what is their origin?

Platelets have a number of functions during the haemostatic response

- *Vasoconstriction (vascular)*: occurs immediately, reducing blood flow to the affected area and allowing contact activation of platelets and coagulation factors
- *Formation of the primary haemostatic plug (platelets)*: this involves the *adhesion* of platelets to collagen, the *release* of contents from its cytoplasmic granules, e.g. serotonin, thromboxane A_2, ADP and fibrinogen, and *aggregation* to other activated platelets
- *Factor binding (coagulation factors)*: platelet membrane phospholipid, though a reaction involving calcium and vitamin K, binds to Factors II, VII, IX and X. It serves to concentrate and coordinate factors into the same area for maximum activation, converting soluble fibrinogen to fibrin clot

Haemostasis depends on interactions between the vessel wall, platelets and coagulation factors (Virchow's triad). Platelets are formed in the bone marrow and released by megakaryocyte fragmentation.

What is von Willebrand's factor?

Von Willebrand's factor (vWF) is a molecule synthesised in megakaryocytes and endothelial cells. It is an essential co-factor for normal platelet adhesion to damaged subendothelium. It also serves as a carrier for Factor VIIIc forming a whole VIII complex, protecting VIIIc from inactivation and clearance.

Which factors are involved in the intrinsic pathway?

The factors of the intrinsic system are Factors VIII (antihaemophilic), IX (Christmas), X (Stuart–Prower), XI (plasma thromboplastin antecedent), XII (Hageman) and XIII (Fletcher and Fitzgerald).

Which factors are involved in the extrinsic pathway?

The factors of the extrinsic system are Factors II (prothrombin), III (tissue), V (labile), VII (proconvertin) and X (Stuart–Prower).

What is the function of vitamin K?

Vitamin K, e.g. phytomenadione, is a fat-soluble vitamin involved in the γ-carboxylation of Factors II, VII, IX and X in the extrinsic pathway. This action allows them to bind to calcium and hence the surface of platelets.

What is the end result of the coagulation cascade?

The end product of the coagulation cascade is the formation of a stable meshwork of cross-linked fibrin around the primary platelet plug. This, therefore, transforms the stable haemostatic plug.

Give some reasons why a surgical patient may develop a coagulopathy?

Causes of a coagulopathy in the surgical patient include

- *Hypothermia*: a cold patient has dysfunctional platelets
- *Massive blood transfusion*: packed red cells do not contain platelets, so a large transfusion leads to a dilutional loss. Also, stored blood rapidly loses the function of the labile Factors V and VIIIc
- *Aspirin*: those with cardiovascular disease may be on aspirin preoperatively. It reduces platelet function by interfering with thromboxane A_2 synthesis
- *Heparin*: in conjunction to its direct effect on clotting, it also causes thrombocytopaenia through an immunological mechanism, e.g. heparin-induced thrombocytopaenia syndrome (HITS)
- *Dextran infusions*: can also affect platelet and coagulation factor function
- *Sepsis*: a cause of DIC
- *Organ damage*: development of post-operative renal or liver failure

How may a coagulopathy be recognised in the surgical patient?

A most common sign of a coagulopathy is unexpected bleeding.

- Bleeding
  - *Preoperative*: bleeding from unusual areas, e.g. venepuncture, cannulation, epistaxis and haematuria from uncomplicated bladder urethral catheterisation
  - *Intraoperative*: persisting microvascular bleeding despite achieving adequate haemostasis
  - *Post-operative*: excessive and continued blood losses in surgical drains, and new-onset purpuric rash representing platelet dysfunction, e.g. HITS

Which tests are used to investigate the coagulopathies?

- Platelet
  - *Count*: ~150–350 × 10^9/L
  - *Function*: bleeding time ~3–8 minutes and adhesion studies, e.g. adrenaline, collagen or ristocetin can be used
- Coagulation times
  - Prothrombin (PT) ~9–15 seconds and is a measure of the extrinsic and common pathways and the degree of warfarin therapy
  - Activated partial thromboplastin (APTT) ~30–40 seconds and is a measure of the intrinsic and common pathways. It is also a measure of heparin therapy
  - Thrombin (TT) ~14–16 seconds and is a measure of the final common pathway
- Individual factor assays
- Plasma D-dimer levels, which measures the fibrin degradation pathway, when testing for DIC

Disseminated intravascular coagulation (DIC)

What is the basic pathophysiology of DIC?

There is pathological activation of the coagulation pathway by damaged tissues which releases cytokines and tissue factors. This is followed by pathologic activation of the fibrinolytic pathway and has a number of effects

- Shock
  - *Hypovolaemic and obstructive*: this produces a low cardiac index, hypotension despite a tachycardia and patients may develop acute kidney injury and ARDS
- Bleeding
  - *Mucosal bleeding and petechial rash*: decreased clotting factors and platelets due to their consumption, manifesting as bleeding from mucosal surfaces
- Thrombosis
  - *Diffuse intravascular thrombosis*: small and large vessel occlusion due to fibrin leading to shock and end-organ failure

How may DIC be triggered?

DIC is indiscriminate and has no demographic as it occurs in all ages, both sexes and equally in all races

Acute DIC

- Severe sepsis
  - Gram-negative
  - Viruses, e.g. HBV, HCV, HIV, CMV in viral haemorrhagic fevers

- ■ Malaria
- Trauma
  - ■ Multiple trauma
  - ■ Burns
  - ■ Hypothermia, e.g. near-drowning
  - ■ Head injury
  - ■ Fat embolism, e.g. long bone fractures
- Organ dysfunction
  - ■ Liver failure
  - ■ Acute pancreatitis (IMRIE >3)
- Obstetric
  - ■ Amniotic fluid embolism
  - ■ Placental abruption
  - ■ Eclampsia
  - ■ Retained foetus
- Immunological
  - ■ Transfusion, e.g. red cells
- Malignancy
  - ■ Disseminated prostatic carcinoma

Chronic DIC

- Vascular
  - ■ Aortic aneurysms
  - ■ Empyemas, e.g. when decortications are required
- Malignancy
  - ■ Adenocarcinoma
- Severe sepsis
  - ■ Osteomyelitis

What type of anaemia may be seen in DIC and why?

Microangiopathic haemolytic anaemia (MAHA) may be seen due to red cell fragmentation caused by fibrin deposition in vessel walls. It can be seen on blood film examination.

What will haematologic investigations show in cases of DIC?

- Plasma D-dimer levels are elevated, indicating activation of the fibrinolytic pathway
- Platelets $<15 \times 10^9$/L due to consumption from activation of the clotting cascade
- Decreased fibrinogen
- Abnormal clotting screen, e.g. ↑PT and ↑APTT in the acute situation
- Reduction in the individual clotting factors

Which blood products are used in the management of DIC?

Platelets and FFP are used to replenish the consumed factors. Packed red cells may also be required if the haemolytic anaemia is severe enough.

Fat embolism syndrome

What is the aetiology of fat embolism syndrome?

Traumatic or non-traumatic critical illness may trigger the fat embolism syndrome

- Long bone fractures, especially of the femur or tibia. More common with closed fractures, possibly since the higher intramedullary pressure forces more fat molecules into the circulation

- Major burns
- Acute pancreatitis, possibly related to pancreatic lipase activity
- Diabetes mellitus
- Orthopaedic procedures, e.g. joint reconstruction
- Decompression sickness
- Cardiopulmonary bypass

What is the pathophysiology of how fat embolism syndrome develops?

There are two main theories

- *Mechanical theory*: this states that the fat droplets gain access to the circulation from the damaged vasculature at the site of fracture. They are carried to the pulmonary vascular bed where they enter the systemic circulation through arteriovenous (AV) shunts. Impaction of these fat emboli in terminal systemic vascular beds produces local ischaemia and tissue injury. This does not explain the non-traumatic causes of this syndrome
- *Biochemical theory*: this explains the syndrome in terms of the release and activation of lipases by stress hormones such as steroid and catecholamines. Lipase hydrolyses circulating platelet bound lipids into free fatty acids (FFA) and glycerol. These FFAs induce pulmonary damage and increase capillary permeability. Platelet activation also increases

5-hydroxy-tryptamine (5-HT), stimulating bronchospasm and vasospasm

What are the clinical features of fat embolism syndrome?
There are a number of clinical features suggesting the syndrome has started. Ninety per cent of these establish themselves within 3 days of the onset of the trigger. Classically, there is the triad of cerebral signs, respiratory insufficiency and a petechial rash

- *Cerebral features*: usually the earliest and most common clinical sign, occurring in up to 90%. Mainly presents as encephalopathy or as a distinct peripheral deficit such as hemiparesis. It is due to
  - Microvessel embolisation of fats and platelet aggregates
  - Activated lipase damaging the lipid-rich platelet cerebral matter
- *Respiratory insufficiency*: seen as tachypnoea and cyanosis 2–3 days following the initial insult. This is due to
  - Pulmonary vascular occlusion by lipid emboli leading to V/Q mismatch and increase shunt
  - Pneumonitis due to mediator release leading to increased capillary permeability and micro-atelectasis. This can lead to pulmonary oedema progressing to the syndrome of acute lung injury or ARDS
  - Superadded pneumonia
- *Petechial rash*: usually seen within 36 hours as a purpura distributed in the area of the chest, axilla, mouth and conjunctiva. It arises as a result of

- Direct embolisation to cutaneous vessels
- Following thrombocytopaenia due to platelet consumption as part of overall pathophysiology

There are a number of less common clinical features that may be seen

- Pyrexia >38°C
- Tachypnoea may be a sign of right ventricular strain
- Retinopathy, following retinal artery embolisation
- Renal impairment, e.g. oliguria, lipiduria and haematuria

Which of these features is pathognomic?

In the right clinical setting, the presence of a petechial rash is pathognomic of the fat embolisation syndrome

What is the role of further investigations in making the diagnosis of fat embolism syndrome?

Given the importance of clinical signs in making the diagnosis of this condition, further investigations have a limited role. They are mainly used in assessing the severity of the condition, and mapping out organ system involvement when planning a management strategy

- *Arterial blood gas (ABG) analysis*: showing a V/Q mismatch, which may be severe enough to produce a Type I respiratory failure
- *Full blood count (FBC)*: a decreased Hb level, e.g. from trauma, may exist, along with a decreased platelet count and an elevated ESR

- *Clotting screen*: this may reveal increased fibrin degradation products, e.g. plasma D-dimer, and elevated APTT and TT
- *Serum electrolytes*: this assesses renal function and reduced serum calcium, due to chelation by circulating lipids
- *Urine*: showing lipiduria
- *Sputum*: shows lipid-laden macrophages and stains for lipid (e.g. by oil red-O)
- *CXR*: showing pulmonary infiltrates (described as a 'snow storm' appearance) or infection
- *CT (head)*: may reveal diffuse white matter petechial haemorrhages consistent with microvascular injury
- *ECG*: showing tachycardia and right ventricular strain (flipped T-waves in the anterior leads)

How is fat embolism syndrome managed?

The main aim of management is supportive measures for the affected organ systems, and the prevention of complications such as renal failure, pulmonary oedema and ARDS.

A number of specific treatments can also be used in an attempt to halt the progression, but these are unproven.

Supportive measures

- *Respiratory support*: using high-flow oxygen and positive end-expiratory pressure (PEEP) if there are signs of ARDS
- *Fluid and electrolyte balance*: if too dry, there will be worsening renal function and acidosis if overloaded, which can exacerbate the presence of pulmonary oedema

- *General measures*: such as DVT prophylaxis, nutritional support and control of sepsis

Specific therapies

- *Albumin solution*: binds to free fatty acids (FFA), but if it leaks through permeable capillaries in the lung, it can make pulmonary oedema worse

The use of ethanol, to reduce lipase activity, Dextran 40, to reduce platelet and red cell aggregation, and heparin, to increase lipase activity to reduce circulating lipids, is controversial.

Can fat embolism syndrome be prevented?
Yes, a number of prophylactic measures may be used to prevent progression to the syndrome

- *Oxygen therapy*: this should be prompt and CPAP can be used to reduce the V/Q deficit by limiting atelectasis
- *Steroids*: there is some evidence that early use of methylprednisolone, e.g. 1.5 mg/kg IV every 8 hours for 6 doses, is beneficial
- *Expedient fracture and immobilisation*: limits the lipid load onto the circulation

What is the prognosis once fat embolism syndrome has been established?
The mortality rate remains at 10–15%, but some of this is reflected in mortality from the underlying cause.

Haemorrhagic shock

What is the definition of shock?

Shock is circulatory failure resulting in inadequate organ perfusion, e.g. cannot meet the metabolic demands. It can be caused by pump failure, e.g. cardiogenic shock (*see* Cardiogenic Shock) or peripheral circulation failure, e.g. hypovolaemia due to haemorrhage.

What types of shock are there and what causes them?

The type of shock may be classified as

- Central
    - *Cardiogenic*: which may be primary, e.g. cardiogenic, or secondary, e.g. pulmonary embolus
- Peripheral
    - *Hypovolaemic*: this is most commonly due to haemorrhage, e.g. trauma, ruptured AAA, and ruptured ectopic pregnancy, fluid loss, e.g. acute pancreatitis (3rd spacing), vomiting secondary to small bowel obstruction, diarrhoea, diuretic abuse and burns, increased insensible losses, e.g. heat exhaustion, persistent pyrexia and drugs
    - *Septic*: from gram-negative organisms generating an endotoxin-induced vasodilatation-producing shock but no signs of infection
    - *Anaphylactic*: a Type I IgE-mediated hypersensitivity reaction, and precipitants include antibiotics, e.g. penicillin

- *Neurogenic*: due to traumatic or iatrogenic, e.g. spinal surgery, injury to the spinal cord causing loss of sympathetic outflow ($\downarrow$HR and $\downarrow$MAP)
- *Obstructive*: due to decreased cardiac output caused by a large acute pulmonary embolus, cardiac tamponade or a tension pneumothorax

Other causes include Addisonian crises and iatrogenic causes, e.g. anaesthetics and antihypertensives. Septic, anaphylactic and neurogenic shock can be grouped together as a distributive form of shock, due to causing a drop in systemic vascular resistance (SVR).

Give some common causes of acute occult bleeding that can give rise to hypovolaemic shock

- Trauma
  - *Fractures (closed)*: of the pelvis (1–3 L), femur (1–2 L) or tibia (0.5–1.0 L)
  - *Thoracic (blunt)*: which injures cardiac, intercostal, pulmonary and other intrathoracic vessels
  - *Abdominal (blunt)*: causing concealed bleeding from the liver or splenic beds
- Spontaneous
  - *Retroperitoneal*: these can occur from ruptured aneurysms, or anticoagulant therapy concealing large volumes of blood
- Obstetric
  - *Perinatal*: due to placental abruption, placenta accreta or retained products

- Iatrogenic
  - *Post-operative*: despite haemostasis being secured intraoperatively, ties and clips can come lose causing exsanguination into a body cavity

Define the haematocrit and what is the normal level?

The haematocrit is the proportion of the blood volume consisting of red cells. If expressed as a fraction of the blood volume, it is 0.4–0.54 in males and 0.37–0.47 in females.

What factors influence the haematocrit?

This is influenced by

- Changes in red cell volume, e.g. due to blood loss
- Changes in plasma volume, e.g. water loss, fluid overload or plasma expansion that occurs in pregnancy

The haematocrit in venous blood is slightly higher than in arterial blood, due to the entry of water and chloride ions into red cells during the chloride shift that occurs with CO_2 carriage.

What are the consequences of a change in the haematocrit?

The implications are

- Changes in the oxygen-carrying capacity of the blood, e.g. polycythaemia at high altitude
- Changes in the viscosity of the blood, which affect the rate and pattern of blood flow in the vascular tree, e.g. thrombotic events

How may the severity of blood loss be classified?

There are four classes depending on the volume lost, percentage of blood lost and clinical signs

- *Class I*: minimal clinical symptoms, blood loss <750 ml (15%), pulse <100 bpm, and blood pressure, pulse pressure, respiratory rate and urine output are all normal. The patient is generally anxious, and can be cool, and crystalloid is the fluid of choice
- *Class II*: the clinical symptoms are more concerning and the patient becomes quite agitated, blood loss 750–1500 ml (15–30%), pulse 100–120 bpm. Despite blood pressure being normal, pulse pressure decreases, respiratory rate increases (20–30/min) and urine output decreases (20–30 ml/h)
- *Class III*: the patient is clinically shocked, having classic signs of inadequate perfusion, blood loss 1500–2000 ml (30–40%), pulse 120–140 bpm, the blood and pulse pressures both decrease, the respiratory rate increases further (30–40/min) and urine output markedly reduces (5–15 ml/h). This blood loss eventually requires a transfusion of red cells. This patient is confused
- *Class IV*: this is immediately life-threatening, requiring urgent surgical intervention to turn off the tap. The patient is cold, pale and loses consciousness, blood loss >2000 ml (>40%), pulse >140 bpm, blood and pulse pressures dramatically decrease, the respiratory rate keeps rising (>40/min) and urine output is non-existent. An immediate transfusion of red cells is required

If a patient starts to decompensate, bradycardia becomes evident. The blood pressure cannot be maintained, demonstrated by a worsening lactic acidosis, despite fluid therapy, e.g. red cells, on ABG analysis due to diminishing organ perfusion. In some cases, mandatory laparotomy is indicated before imaging.

Why do decompensating patients often become bradycardic?

This is due to

- Reflexes
  - *Depressor reflex*: diminished ventricular filling deforms the ventricular wall, activating myocardial vagal C-fibres to produce a bradycardia in the context of blood loss. It perversely exerts a myocardial protective effect by reducing myocardial oxygen demand

Outline the autonomic response to blood loss

The autonomic response is due to decreased venous return (preload) secondary to hypovolaemia, which causes a drop in cardiac output and arterial pressure by the Frank–Starling mechanism

- Reflexes
  - *Baroreceptor*: stimulates sympathetic activity producing a compensatory tachycardia, increased stroke volume and peripheral vessel constriction ($\uparrow$SVR). This increases the cardiac output and maintains blood pressure
- Hormones

- *Catecholamines*: the adrenal medulla is stimulated by pain and injury and releases hormones to cause peripheral vessel constriction, e.g. noradrenaline (↑SVR)
- *Mineralocorticoids*: the adrenal cortex releases hormones to stimulate salt and water retention, e.g. cortisol to increase the blood pressure

The reduction in the circulating volume, and increased sympathetic activity, stimulates renin release from the macula densa of the juxtaglomerular apparatus of the kidney, e.g. renin–angiotensin–aldosterone (RAA) cascade. A resultant increase in salt and water retention helps to restore circulating volume over several hours.

What are the two major types of abdominal trauma and which organs are most affected?

The two types of injury are blunt and penetrating. The most commonly injured organs are liver, spleen and kidney.

How might suspected intra-abdominal haemorrhage be investigated?

This usually involves

- *US*: focused assessment with sonography in trauma (FAST). It has a sensitivity, specificity and accuracy comparable to diagnostic peritoneal lavage (DPL) and is non-invasive and extremely quick
- *CT*: this can be used if FAST is compromised due to obesity, subcutaneous air or previous abdominal operations, and a

whole trauma serious of images, e.g. head, neck, chest, abdomen, pelvis, can be obtained

What is the basic management of blood loss?
All cases require immediate ABCDE assessment, appropriate laboratory and radiological investigations to enable adequate fluid resuscitation (including blood), cross-matching for theatre and evaluation of the underlying cause, e.g. permissive hypotension in ruptured AAA to guide endovascular or surgical approaches. Management of circulation and haemorrhage control includes

- *Vascular access*: the Hagen–Poiseuille equation states fluid flow through a tube is proportional to the 4th power of its radius but inversely proportional to its length. A short fat tube, e.g. a 14-G, in both ante-cubital fossae, not a thin long tube, e.g. a CVP line, is required
- *Fluids*: adequate fluid resuscitation using either crystalloids or colloids increases the blood pressure by improving venous return, stroke volume and the cardiac output. However, only a transfusion of red cells (*see* Fluid Therapy) improves the oxygen-carrying capacity of the blood
- *Monitoring response*: the body's response to resuscitation should be measured, and a CVP line, to assess central circulatory volumes, and a urinary catheter, as an indirect measure of renal function, are useful tools
- *Mechanical compression*: if there is an open site of bleeding, digital pressure or the use of splints and tourniquets can be used

Ultimately, following resuscitation and stabilisation, surgical intervention may be required to gain definitive control of the bleeding e.g. craniotomy, thoracotomy, laparotomy, fracture fixation. In cases of trauma, the ATLS® protocol should be adhered to, and CCrISP® in critically unwell surgical patients.

Procedures

Arterial lines: intra-arterial blood pressure monitoring

What is the purpose of an arterial line?

This serves two purposes

- *Intra-arterial blood pressure (IABP) monitoring*: this provides continuous beat to beat blood pressure, e.g. patients requiring inotropic support and complex neurosurgical, cardiothoracic and vascular operations (*see* Blood Pressure Monitoring)
- *Arterial blood gas (ABG) analysis*: this is useful to aspirate blood for ABG analysis preventing multiple stab attempts and, therefore, decreasing the risk of false aneurysmal formation, double punctures and infection

Which vessels may be used for arterial line?

- Common
  - Radial artery
- Uncommon
  - Ulnar artery
  - Femoral artery

**What are the pre-procedure checks required for a
safe insertion?**

All indications for an arterial line require ABCDE assessment,
reviewing of laboratory and necessary radiological
investigations, and assembly of all required equipment. The
most important clinical test is Allen's test to determine the
presence of adequate collateral flow in the ulnar artery (*see*
Blood Pressure Monitoring) if radial artery cannulation is
sought.

- Laboratory
  - *Prothrombin time (PT)*: e.g. in patients on warfarin
    anticoagulation, despite there being no evidence that
    deranged clotting exacerbates post-procedure bleeding, it
    is good medical practice to check
  - *Platelet count*: in patients at risk of prolonged bleeding
    due to haematological diseases, e.g. haemophilia, it is
    prudent to check

Written informed consent from the patient should be
obtained to both the arterial line and appropriate local
anaesthetic. Patients should be transferred to an HDU bed to
permit cardiorespiratory monitoring throughout the
procedure.

**List the equipment needed and outline the
steps for insertion**

An assembly of equipment is needed and includes an arterial
cannula, arterial giving set, 500 ml 0.9% NaCl bag, pressure bag

(to pressurise the saline to 300 mmHg), connecting tubing, transducer, amplifier and electrical recording equipment, all opened in an aseptic non-touch sterile technique.

- *Positioning*: the patient is can be positioned sitting in a recumbent position but the wrist might be extended and stabilised ensuring the artery is more superficial
- *Marking*: a readily palpable radial artery is chosen, e.g. there might be a history of radial artery harvesting for coronary artery bypass grafting which may prevent the use of the opposite side
- *Prep and drape*: following careful hand-washing, the skin is cleaned from shoulder to fingertips using Betadine® and the patient is draped exposing the designated area
- *Infiltration of local anaesthetic (LA)*: e.g. 2 ml 1% lignocaine (lidocaine) is used to make a small wheal over the skin using an orange needle before 10–15 ml is used to progressively infiltrate the subcutaneous layers
- *Insertion of arterial line*: once palpated, the line is inserted according to the Seldinger technique (*see* pp. 151–152). The introducing needle and guide wire is directed proximally at 30° to the skin and should be passed freely, never forced
- *Security*: it is sutured in place using silk
- *Transducer*: pre-procedure it is zeroed and placed at heart level. The saline bag is pressurised to prevent back flow from the cannula, and enable a continuous slow flushing system of 3–4 ml/h to prevent clot formation

What are the complications of an arterial line insertion?

The complications include

- *Exsanguination*: haemorrhage occurs if there are leaks in the system
- *Occlusion*: this includes partial occlusion, e.g. due to large cannula widths and multiple attempts, and occurs in 1.5–35%, and complete occlusion, e.g. due to pre-existing arterial disease, vasopressors and digital ischaemia, and can occur in <0.1%
- *Infection*: this is particularly rare (complications ∼0.13%) and is identified by erythema around the insertion site, a tender radium and developing sepsis not attributable to other causes
- *Embolism*: this can be due to the introduction of air or thrombus formation and subsequent embolic disease following partial occlusion

Other complications include pseudoaneurysms and iatrogenic permanent hand damage due to drug administration. Consequently, arterial lines should never be used as a route to administer drugs and should be labelled in red.

Contraindications include digital vasculitis and patients who are going to have the radial artery on that side harvested as a conduit for bypass surgery.

How do arterial lines work?

The column of saline in the arterial giving set transmits the pressure changes associated with changes in blood pressure to the diaphragm in the transducer. This produces an electrical signal which is displayed as an arterial waveform.

What is meant by the term 'swing in the arterial line' during continuous measurements, and what is its significance?

This refers to a variation of the amplitude in the arterial tracing during the respiratory cycle. It is an indicator that the patient is under filled and requires more fluid resuscitation.

Central access: central lines

What is the purpose of a central venous catheter (CVC)?

These act as an adjunct to cardiovascular treatment and management and have several purposes

- Short term
  - *Central venous pressure (CVP)*: measurement and continuous monitoring of the CVP
  - *Pulmonary artery flotation catheter*: this is useful to evaluate direct, e.g. pulmonary artery capillary wedge pressure (PACWP), and to calculate derived, e.g. stroke volume, measures of cardiovascular function (*see* Chapter 6, Pulmonary Artery Catheters)
  - *Fluid balance*: it can be used to guide fluid resuscitation and patients prone to failures of the heart, lungs and kidneys, and during complex neurosurgical, cardiothoracic and vascular operations

- *Drug administration*: a large central line is useful for administering drugs irritant to veins, e.g. amiodarone or inotropes
- *Haemodialysis*: can be a conduit for renal replacement therapy
- *Cardiac pacing*: if transcutaneous pacing fails, then transvenous pacing can be rapidly conducted through an indwelling central line
- Long term
  - *Venous access (blood sampling)*: aspiration of blood substitutes the need for venepuncture in the compromised patient; however, lines should be regularly tested for line sepsis
  - *Chemotherapy*: cytotoxic agents and other long-term drugs can be administered
  - *Total parenteral nutrition (TPN)*: provides a useful route to feed patients unable to tolerate oral intake or are needing nutritional fortification (*see* Chapter 5, Burns)

To reduce infection, these lines may be tunnelled beneath the skin for a short distance before entering the vein. Patency is ensured by regular heparin saline flushes.

Which vessels may be used for central venous access?
- Common
  - Internal jugular vein (most common)
  - Subclavian vein
  - Femoral vein

- Uncommon
  - Axilliary vein
  - Cephalic vein
  - External jugular vein

What is the central venous pressure (CVP) and how may it be determined?

This is the pressure in the right atrium (right atrial filling pressure). It may be estimated clinically by examining the jugular venous pulse at the root of the neck or measured directly by inserting a CVC.

What is the normal value for the CVP?

The normal value ranges between 2 and 6 mmHg or between 5 and 12 cmH$_2$O.

How useful is it as a measure of the circulating volume?

The absolute value of the CVP is not as useful as its response to a 200–300 ml fluid challenge (over 1–3 min) in determining filling. In some critically ill patients (mainly cardiac and pulmonary diseases) where the myocardial compliance is affected, the CVP reading provides an inaccurate estimate of the volume state. Thus, the reading has to be interpreted in the light of other physiological parameters (*see* following diagram).

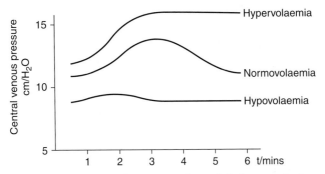

Figure 3.11 Adapted with permission from *Clinical Surgery in General,* 3rd edn. Edited by Kirk, Mansfield and Cochrane (1999), p. 357. Published by Churchill Livingstone, ISBN 0443062196.

What are the pre-procedure checks required for a safe insertion?

All indications for a central line require ABCDE assessment, reviewing of laboratory and radiological investigations, and assembly of all required equipment.

- Laboratory
  - *Prothrombin time (PT)*: e.g. in patients on warfarin anticoagulation, it is good medical practice to check, despite there being no evidence that deranged clotting exacerbates post-procedure bleeding
  - *Platelet count*: it is prudent to check in patients at risk of prolonged bleeding due to haematological diseases, e.g. haemophilia
- Radiological

- *CXR*: this is mandatory due to the risk of iatrogenic injury to the lung and pleural reflections, e.g. hyperinflation in COPD, and presence of pneumothoraces, haemothoraces
- Microbiology
  - *Sepsis*: the presence of infection overlying the insertion site is a relative contraindication due to the risk of line sepsis

Written informed consent from the patient should be obtained (where possible) to both the central line and appropriate local anaesthetic (and light sedation if necessary). Patients should be transferred to an HDU bed to permit cardiorespiratory monitoring throughout the procedure, but it should ideally be performed in theatre under ultrasonic guidance.

List the equipment needed and outline the steps for insertion

An assembly of equipment is needed and includes a sterile pack, drapes, gauze swabs, sterile gloves, cap and mask, antiseptic solution, local anaesthetic, catheter, universal containers, the ultrasound probe in a sterile sheath and dressings, all opened in an aseptic non-touch sterile technique.

- *Positioning*: the patient is positioned head down and feet up, e.g. the Trendelenburg position, to increase vein size for internal jugular or subclavian vein approach
- *Marking*: surface anatomical landmarks are identified before 2D ultrasound (US) is used to identify the chosen vein (*see* below). The internal jugular may be approached as it lies deep to the two heads of the sternocleidomastoid, but if for

subclavian cannulation, the approach is infra-clavicular (2 cm below the mid-point of the clavicle). The artery is usually medial to the internal jugular and is not compressible

- *Prep and drape*: following scrubbing and gowning, the skin is cleaned from clavicle to pelvis using Betadine® and the patient is draped exposing the designated area
- *Infiltration of local anaesthetic (LA)*: e.g. 2 ml 1% lignocaine (lidocaine) is used to make a small wheal over the skin using an orange needle before 10–15 ml is used to progressively infiltrate the subcutaneous layers using a green needle (but not deep to the subcutaneous tissues)
- *Insertion of CVC*: is conducted according to the Seldinger technique. The introducing needle and guide wire is directed inferiorly parallel to the sagittal plane at 30° to the skin and deep to the clavicle pointing to the jugular notch. It is advanced under US guidance while applying negative pressure to the syringe until a flash of blood is seen
- *Security*: it should be sutured in place using silk
- *Collection*: some blood is sent for routine haematology, biochemistry and microbiology analysis

Surface anatomical landmarks for the internal jugular vein runs from the lobule of the ear to the medial end of the clavicle. It then lies between the two heads of the sternocleidomastoid muscle. Behind the sterno-clavicular joint it unites with the subclavian vein to form the right brachiocephalic vein. This joins the left brachiocephalic behind the right 1st costal cartilage to form the superior vena cava (SVC). This passes vertically down and pierces the pericardium at the level of the 2nd costal cartilage, entering the right atrium behind the 3rd costal cartilage.

Ultrasound (2D) guidance is recommended for central line insertion in both the elective and emergency situation. It precisely identifies the target vein, potential anatomical variations and intraluminal thrombosis.

A chest radiograph is taken at the end of the procedure to ensure a correct position and exclude a pneumothorax or haemothorax.

What is the Seldinger technique?

This technique of cannulation involves the use of a guide wire passed through an introducing needle. A wider bore cannula (dual or tri-lumen) is then passed over the wire after removal of the introducing needle (then the wire is removed). These principles can also be applied to other procedures, e.g. paracentesis or percutaneous tracheostomy.

What are the complications of a central line insertion?

The complications include

- *Pleural*: this can have a rapid onset, e.g. pneumothorax, or be delayed, e.g. haemothorax
- *Venous*: air can be introduced resulting in an air embolism (>20 ml), thrombogenic formation, and emboli can occur around the line tip
- *Arterial*: inadvertent cannulation of a surrounding arterial structure can result in local haematoma formation,

haemothorax and exsanguination, e.g. the bleeding from the subclavian artery requires emergency vascular control and repair
- *Lymphatic*: the thoracic duct can be injured leading to a chylothorax
- *Cardiac*: perforation of the right atria can occur leading to cardiac tamponade, and arrhythmias can develop warranting continuous ECG monitoring throughout
- *Sepsis*: this can be caused by the introduction of skin microbes during insertion or repeated use of aspirating blood

Other complications include malposition and coiling of the catheter and catheter embolism.

What are the indications for removal of a central line?
- Cessation of cardiac support in the form of inotropes and vasopressors
- Resolution of an acute presentation and return to normal pre-admission baseline parameters
- Discontinuation of renal replacement therapy
- Line sepsis
- Discharge home

In which two ways may the information from a central line be presented?
The information can be presented as a continuous waveform using a transducer attached to an oscilloscope, or it can be measured intermittently by using a manometer system at the bedside.

Which formula governs the rate of flow through tubes, and how does this affect the use of a central line in fluid resuscitation?

Simply put, flow is defined by the Hagen–Poiseuille formula which states that

$$\text{Flow through a rigid tube} = \frac{Pr^4 \pi}{8\eta L}$$

Thus, the greatest flow can be achieved with short wide tubes. The radius of the tube has the greatest impact, since the flow is proportional to the 4th power of the radius. Central lines are not the most effective for rapid fluid administration, because of their length and radius.

Bibliography

American College of Surgeons. Shock. In *Advanced Trauma Life Support® (ATLS®)*, 9th edn. Chicago, IL, American College of Surgeons; 2012: Chapter 3.

Hebballi R, Swanevelder J. Diagnosis and management of aortic dissection. *Continuing Education in Anaesthesia, Critical Care & Pain Journal.* 2009;9(1): 14–18.

Hignett R, Stephens R. Practical procedures: radial arterial lines. *British Journal of Hospital Medicine.* 2006;67(5): M3–M5.

Norfolk D. *Handbook of Transfusion Handbook*, 5th edn. Norwich, Joint United Kingdom (UK) Blood Transfusion and Tissue Transplantation Services Professional Advisory Committee, 2014.

Resuscitation Council (UK). Peri-arrest arrhythmias. In *Advanced Life Support*, 6th edn. London, Resuscitation Council (UK) Trading Ltd; 2011: Chapter 11.

Royal College of Surgeons of England. Cardiovascular disorders, diagnosis and management. In *Care of the Critically Ill Surgical Patient (CCrISP®)*, 3rd edn. London, Royal College of Surgeons of England; 2010: Chapter 6.

Royal College of Surgeons of England. Shock and haemorrhage. In *Care of the Critically Ill Surgical Patient (CCrISP®)*, 3rd edn. London, Royal College of Surgeons of England; 2010: Chapter 7.

SIGN Clinical Guideline 77. Postoperative management in adults: a practical guide to postoperative care for clinical staff. Chapter 3 cardiovascular management. *Scottish Intercollegiate Guidelines Network (SIGN)*. 2004;77: 11–19.

SIGN Clinical Guideline 129. Antithrombotics: indications and management. *Scottish Intercollegiate Guidelines Network (SIGN)*. 2013; 129: 1–19.

Chapter 4

Disability (neurological evalution)

Assessment

Neurological assessment

Which basic investigations may be used in assessing neurological function?

Following basic clinical examination of the central and peripheral nervous system, investigations may include

Non-invasive

- *Glasgow Coma Scale (GCS)*: this is a clinical assessment of a patient's ability to see a threat, communicate a threat and generate a motor response to defend itself. The maximum score is 15 and the lowest score is 3
  - *Eyes (Max 4)*: spontaneous eye opening (4), opens eyes to a vocal stimulus (3), opens eyes to a painful stimulus (2), no eye opening (1)
  - *Voice (Max 5)*: coherent speech (5), confused speech (4), inappropriate words (3), sounds (2), no sounds (1)
  - *Motor (Max 6)*: obeys commands (6), localises to pain (5), withdraws from pain (4), flexor decorticate response (3), extensor decerebrate response (2), no response (1)

- *Radiology*: high-resolution CT – head, MRI – head
- *Transcranial Doppler (TCD)*: measures blood velocity in large cerebral arteries, e.g. middle cerebral
- *Electroencephalograph (EEG)*: measures electrical signals generated in central neural tissue

The assessment of the GCS is extremely important, and must be measured again if unsure until a precise score has been determined. Of the three components, a drop in the motor score is most prognostic.

NB. The term 'scale' regards the observed description of each component, e.g. 'spontaneous eye opening', whereas the term 'score' is simply the summation of the points score in each section, e.g. 12. The term 'score' in isolation from the term 'scale', simply provides a number but no clinical context, as a score of 12 can be composed of many different variables when accessing eyes, voice and motor.

Invasive

- *Lumbar puncture (LP)*: is used to extract cerebrospinal fluid (CSF) for visual, microbiological, cytological and biochemical analysis
- *Intracranial pressure monitoring (ICP)*: e.g. ICP bolt, is useful to measure actual, and fluctuations in the, intracranial pressure to predict deterioration in patients where GCS cannot be measured
- *Digital subtraction angiography (DSA)*: this is the gold standard diagnostic procedure for investigating cerebral ischaemia, but its complications include stroke

- *Positron emission tomography (PET)*: is used to evaluate cerebral blood flow or cerebral metabolism

Basic concepts

Analgesia

What class of analgesics are there?

There are three analgesic steps according to the World Health Organisation (WHO)

- *Step 1 (non-opioid)*: mild pain, e.g. paracetamol or non-steroidal anti-inflammatory drugs (NSAIDs)
- *Step 2 (weak opioid)*: moderate pain, e.g. codeine or tramadol. Step 1 analgesics can be added
- *Step 3 (strong opioid)*: severe pain, e.g. morphine, pethidine. Step 1 and Step 2 analgesics can be added

How may analgesics be administered?

The common routes of administration are

Enteral

- *Oral (PO)*: this includes sublingual and rectal administration and is used to administer Step 1 and some Step 2 analgesics

Parenteral

- *Intravenous (IV)*: includes IV infusions and patient-controlled analgesia (PCA) and is used to administer some Step 1, e.g. paracetamol, some Step 2, e.g. tramadol, and all Step 3 analgesics, e.g. morphine

- *Intramuscular (IM)*: this is used to administer some Step 2 analgesics
- *Intranasal (IN)*: for opiates in the paediatric setting
- *Intrathecal (IT)*: is used to administer epidural analgesia during some thoracic surgery
- *Inhalation (INH)*: can be useful in the emergency setting, e.g. nitrous oxide, in manipulating fractures in the Emergency Department
- *Transcutaneous (TC)*: can be used to apply Step 3 analgesics for chronic pain, e.g. fentanyl patch

Give some examples of the opiates in common use. Which are the synthetic and which are the non-synthetic agents?
The commonly used opiates are

- *Non-synthetic*: morphine, codeine (10% of this is metabolised to morphine)
- *Semi-synthetic*: diamorphine, dihydrocodeine
- *Synthetic*: pethidine, fentanyl

Which receptor do opiate analgesics act on?
Opiates mostly activate the μ-receptor to generate their effects, but some also have efficacy at the κ- and γ-receptors.

What are the systemic effects of the opiates?
The effects of the opiates are

- *Systemic*: they are good for moderate to severe pain of any cause and modality. However, they are less effective for neuropathic pain, e.g. phantom limb pain or allodynia (pain from a non-painful stimulus)

- *Respiratory (depression)*: blunting of the chemoreceptor response to rising $PaCO_2$. Also causes suppression of the cough reflex, both of which encourage sputum retention, atelectasis and pneumonia in the critically ill
- *Neurological (sedation)*: there is a reduction in the level of consciousness at higher doses, so beware in those with head injuries
- *Gastrointestinal (nausea, vomiting, reduced motility)*: following stimulation of the chemoreceptor trigger zone in the area postrema and reduced motility can lead to constipation
- *Psychiatric (euphoria, dependence, tolerance)*: the initial euphoria can lead to a progressively reduced effect from the same dose of drug, increased tolerance and dependence
- *Immunological*: histamine release from mast cells produces pruritis and reduced systemic vascular resistance

Why is morphine not advocated for use in abdominal pain of biliary origin?

Morphine increases the tone of the sphincter of Oddi (as well as other sphincteric muscles), simultaneous to stimulating contraction of the gallbladder. Therefore, it can exacerbate biliary pain.

Which drug is given for opiate overdose? What is the mechanism of action?

Naloxone may be used to reverse the effects of opioids. This is a short-acting μ-receptor antagonist. NB. Because of its short duration of action the effects of the opioids may return after an initial reversal.

What are the therapeutic effects of paracetamol (acetaminophen)?

This is an analgesic and anti-pyretic with minimal anti-inflammatory properties.

By what mechanism does overdose cause liver injury?

The subsequent liver injury is due to paracetamol metabolism. Normally it is conjugated in the liver and produces a small amount of the toxic metabolite N-acetylbenzoquinoneimine. Binding to hepatic glutathione renders this metabolite harmless. With overdose, glutathione is depleted, leading to hepatocyte injury. Acetylcysteine, the drug used to treat overdose, is a glutathione precursor.

How do non-steroidal anti-inflammatory drugs (NSAIDs) work?

These agents act to reduce prostaglandin (PG) formation by the inhibition of the enzyme cyclooxygenase (COX), which acts on arachidonic acid. This leads to a modification of the inflammatory reaction and its effects on the stimulating nociception.

What are NSAIDs systemic side effects?

The systemic side effects of these agents include

- *Gastrointestinal*: dyspepsia, gastritis and peptic ulceration. There is direct stimulation of acid secretion by the gastric

parietal cells, with reduced bicarbonate and mucus
production

- *Renal*: may precipitate acute kidney injury, especially in
  those with pre-existing chronic kidney disease, dehydration,
  hypotension or co-existent nephrotoxic pharmacological
  therapy. It also leads to salt and water retention
- *Coagulopathy*: inhibition of platelet thromboxane A_2
  production leads to their reduced ability to aggregate and
  form the primary platelet plug. This is a permanent effect,
  and is reversed only when new platelets are formed
- *Bronchospasm*: the inhibition of COX leads to arachidonic
  acid being metabolised down the pathway of leucotriene
  formation, which induces bronchospasm

How is renal injury precipitated?

There is inhibition of compensatory PG_{I2} and PG_{E2} formation
that occurs during situations of reduced renal perfusion. These
prostaglandins normally promote vasodilatation during such
situations, offsetting the development of acute tubular
necrosis.

What local anaesthetic techniques are available
for pain relief?

The local anaesthetic techniques available are

- *Local nerve blocks*: such as the 3 in 1 block of the lateral
  cutaneous, femoral and obturator nerves that can be used
  for fractured neck of femur. Other examples include

intercostal blocks following chest injury and paravertebral blocks, e.g. post-thoracic surgery

- *Epidural and spinal block*: the former is more popular because of its longer duration of action and reduced systemic adverse effects

When is epidural analgesia commonly employed?

Epidural analgesia is commonly used in the post-operative setting, being especially useful in situations where pain may compromise respiratory function, e.g. thoracic or upper abdominal surgery.

Why is epidural analgesia's use limited in the critical care setting?

- *Sepsis*: the patient may be septic or have a local infection, both of which contraindicate the use of an epidural
- *Coagulopathy*: epidurals must not be inserted in the presence of a coagulopathy
- *Hypovolaemia*: if hypovolaemia is present, this can lead to decompensated hypotension if an epidural is used

Due to these attendant contraindications and risks, in most situations it does require the patient to be fully informed and consented

What are the potential systemic effects of this form of analgesia?

Some of the systemic effects of epidurals include

- *Hypotension*: due to block of the sympathetic outflow causing peripheral vasodilatation, and a reduction in cardiac output may occur due to a reduction in venous return
- *General*: attenuation of the surgical stress response
- *Respiratory*: reduction of the functional residual capacity (FRC)
- *Coagulopathy*: reduction of post-operative deep venous thrombosis (DVT) due to a number of causes, including the concomitant use of IV fluids used to support the arterial pressure

Complex concepts

Cerebral physiology: basic principles

What is the volume of the cerebrospinal fluid (CSF)?
140–150 ml.

Where is CSF produced, and at what rate?
Roughly 70% of CSF is produced by the choroid plexus of the lateral, 3rd and 4th ventricles. The remaining 30% comes directly from the vessels lining the ventricular walls. It is produced at a rate of 0.20–0.35 ml/min ($\sim$500 ml/day).

Briefly describe the circulation of CSF
The circulation of CSF can be considered to begin in the lateral ventricles, coursing caudally into the 3rd ventricle through the interventricular foramen of Monro. From this reservoir it then enters the 4th ventricle through the aqueduct of Sylvius. Some fluid continues down into the central canal of the spinal cord,

but the majority flows into the subarachnoid space of the
spinal cord via the central foramen of Magendie, or the two
lateral foramina of Luschka. After going around the spinal
cord, it enters the cranial cavity through the foramen magnum,
and flows around the brain in the subarachnoid space.

What are the arachnoid villi composed of?
The arachnoid villi are formed from a fusion of arachnoid
membrane and the endothelium of the dural venous sinus that
it has bulged into.

Where is CSF absorbed?
Up to 80% of CSF is absorbed at the arachnoid villi, and 20% is
absorbed in the spinal nerve roots.

What structures form the blood–brain barrier (BBB)?
The BBB is a histological and physiological boundary between
the blood and the CSF. It is formed from two types of special
anatomical arrangement

- *Tight junctions*: these occur in-between the endothelial cells
  of the cerebral capillaries
- *Astrocytic foot processes*: these are applied to the basal
  membranes of the cerebral capillaries

What substances can pass through the BBB?
The BBB is permeable to lipids, lipid-soluble molecules, e.g.
opiates and general anaesthetics, respiratory gases and
glucose. Chronically, it is also permeable to protons (H^+).

Which parts of the brain lie outside of the BBB?

Three main areas lie outside the BBB and include

- *Neurohypophysis*: this is the posterior lobe of the pituitary gland, which produces vasopressin (ADH) and oxytocin
- *Circumventricular organs*: these are situated around the 3rd and 4th ventricles, which include the supraoptic crest, area postrema and tuber cinereum

The median eminence of the hypothalamus is also located outside the BBB.

Which pathologies can affect the integrity of the BBB?

The integrity of the BBB is compromised by infection, tumours, trauma and ischaemia.

What is the cerebral blood flow?

The total flow is $\sim$750 ml/min ($\sim$15%) of the cardiac output. This equates to a cerebral blood flow of $\sim$50 ml/100 g of tissue.

How does cerebral blood flow vary with the arterial pressure?

This cerebral blood flow remains constant between a systemic systolic blood pressure of 50 and 150 mmHg, due to local auto-regulation of flow.

What is the mechanism of auto-regulation?

There are two main factors that allow the cerebral blood flow to remain constant despite variations in the driving pressure

- *Myogenic*: an increase in the wall tension caused by a rise in the mean arterial pressure stimulates a reactive contraction of smooth muscle cells. This increases the vascular resistance, keeping the flow constant
- *Metabolic (vasodilator 'washout')*: if blood flow is momentarily increased by a sudden rise in arterial pressure, locally produced vasodilator substances are washed out, leading to increased vascular resistance, and so a return of flow back to the normal
- *Neurogenic*: sympathetic stimulation can affect arteriolar tone, and nitric oxide (NO) released by parasympathetic fibres may also play a role

What other factors regulate the cerebral blood flow?

Blood flow is affected by several factors

- *Carbon dioxide (CO_2)*: has a profound and reversible effect on cerebral blood flow, e.g. hypercapnia causes marked dilation of cerebral arterioles and increases blood flow, but hypocapnia causes constriction and decreased blood flow. This is due to the effect of extracellular H^+ on vascular smooth muscle
- *Oxygen (O_2)*: the brain has a very high metabolic demand for oxygen. Therefore, acute hypoxia, e.g. $PaO_2 < 6.7$ kPa is a potent dilator in the cerebral circulation that produces marked increases in cerebral blood flow

This has considerations for managing high intracranial pressure through the manipulation of CO_2.

Define the cerebral perfusion pressure (CPP)

The cerebral perfusion pressure (CPP) is defined as the difference between mean arterial pressure (MAP) and intracranial pressure (ICP)

$$CPP = MAP - ICP$$

It must remain above ~70 mmHg for the brain tissue to be adequately perfused. Processes that increase the ICP, e.g. tumours, oedema, bleeds, blockage of CSF circulation, compromise the CPP, contributing to subsequent ischaemia, infraction and necrosis.

What is the Cushing reflex?

This is mixed vagal and sympathetic stimulation that occurs in response to an elevated ICP. It leads to hypertension to maintain the CPP and a resultant bradycardia.

Cerebral pathophysiology: basic principles

What is the Monro–Kellie doctrine?

This considers the cranial cavity as a rigid sphere containing non-compressible contents, e.g. brain, blood and CSF. Consequently, an increase of one of these contents necessarily decreases one of the others to a varying degree.

Draw a graph showing the relationship of the intracranial pressure (ICP) to the intracranial volume. What does this show?

This shows the changing nature of the compliance of the intracranial contents with increases in the ICP. A small rise in volume leads to little rise in the ICP due to a relatively higher intracranial compliance. At higher volumes there is an exponential rise in the ICP as compliance decreases due to volume overload. This critical point of ICP decompensation differs among individuals.

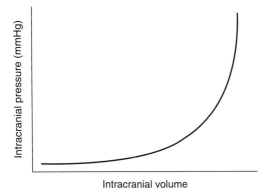

Figure 4.1 The relationship between the intracranial volume and intracranial pressure.

Give some basic causes of a raised ICP

- *CSF*: an increase in volume, e.g. hydrocephalus, can occur due to increased production, decreased absorption or blockage in the intraventricular and communicating channels
- *Blood*: this is usually due to intracranial bleeding, e.g. subdural (SDH), extradural (EDH), subarachnoid (SAH) and intracerebral causes (stroke)
- *Brain*: a space-occupying lesion, apart from blood and CSF. Includes tumours, cerebral oedema and idiopathic intracranial hypertension (IIH)

What are the signs and symptoms of a raised ICP?

Some of the signs and symptoms of a raised ICP include

- *Headache*: often worse in the morning due to being in a recumbent position, decreasing caudal drainage
- *Nausea and vomiting*: often worse in the morning
- *Reduced GCS*: may manifest as simple drowsiness. This is an important sign, as its significance may be missed
- *Papilloedema*: a definitive sign of a chronically raised ICP as it takes 2 weeks to develop, and is bilateral. The pressure is transmitted along the subarachnoid space of the optic nerve

Why should the ICP be controlled? What techniques are available?

There are two main reasons why the ICP should be controlled

- A high ICP can lead to cerebral herniation
- A high ICP causes a reduction of the cerebral perfusion pressure (since CPP = MAP − ICP)

There are a number of techniques used to reduce the ICP using conservative rather than surgical measures

- *Positioning*: tilting the end of the bed 20–30° (head up) and loosening of tracheal tapes and neck collars to aid cerebral venous drainage
- *Fluid restriction*: to prevent cerebral oedema, e.g. a life-threatening complication of managing diabetic ketoacidosis (DKA)

- *Diuretics*: e.g. mannitol, which is an osmotic diuretic given at a dose of 0.25–1.00 g/kg over 20–30 minutes. It rapidly decreases ICP and is useful before hospital transfers
- *Controlled ventilation*: keeping the PaCO_2 between 4.0 and 4.5 kPa enables CO_2 to control the degree of intracranial vasodilatation
- *Drainage*: this can be done by direct tapping of CSF from a ventricular catheter
- *Barbiturates*: e.g. thiopentone, if the ICP is resistant to the above measures
- *Surgery*: a decompressive craniectomy can be performed for malignant increases in ICP refractory to optimal medical therapy. It is controversial and has gained widespread scrutiny

NB. Steroids are helpful in reducing the swelling around cerebral tumours but not in situations of cerebral trauma. However, they are useful in cases of spinal injury.

What is the most important and life-threatening complication of raised ICP?

The most significant complication is cerebral herniation. This can lead to rapid onset of coma, respiratory failure and death.

What varieties of brain herniation are there, and how may they manifest themselves?

The clue to cerebral herniation is what is herniating, where it is herniating and what is being compressed. Some of the types of brain herniation include

- *Subfalcine*: the cingulate gyrus herniates beneath the falx cerebri between the two supratentorial compartments. The anterior cerebral artery (ACA) is compressed
- *Tonsillar*: leading to displacement of the cerebellar tonsils through the foramen magnum. The medulla oblongata is compressed, crushing cardiorespiratory centres leading to respiratory depression
- *Transtentorial*: the uncus of the temporal lobe passes through the tentorial hiatus (tentorial incisura), compressing the midbrain and posterior cerebral artery (PCA)

Herniation can lead to a number of effects; transtentorial herniation can lead to ipsilateral compression of the oculomotor nerve (CN III) and pyramidal tract running in the midbrain. This is clinically manifest as an ipsilateral dilated pupil and a contralateral hemiparesis. Displacement of the PCA may produce visual-field defects with transtentorial herniation, and pressure on the brainstem stimulates Cheyne–Stokes respiration and the Cushing reflex. An exponential rise in the ICP is produced as flow of the CSF is suddenly occluded by the herniated brain.

Name a false localising sign – why does this occur?
The classical false localising sign is an abducent (CN VI) nerve palsy, i.e. the inability to abduct the eye. This falsely points to the abducent motor nucleus as being the site of the lesion. In reality it results from herniation producing kinking of the 6th nerve as it runs a long intracranial course.

When would you perform a CT scan?

If a patient develops an unexpected drop in GCS and has focal neurological changes from their baseline on clinical examination, a CT head is performed. Other indications include

- *Signs*: persisting neurological signs as a sudden change from normal and change in GCS
- *Symptoms*: persisting headache and signs indicating meningism, e.g. nausea, vomiting, photophobia, neck stiffness

Other indications include a history of trauma and suspicion of a basal skull fracture, e.g. otorrhoea, rhinorrhoea, subconjunctival haemorrhage, periorbital haematoma, Battle's sign or a penetrating injury.

Briefly outline a strategy for the management of a neurologically compromised patient

This depends on the underlying history, mechanism, associated co-morbidities and findings on CT scan, and can be simply classified according to the three basic causes of a raised ICP

- *CSF*: if there is isolated hydrocephalus, e.g. no bleed, space-occupying lesion or herniation, a ventriculoperitoneal (VP) shunt can be placed, but in the acute situation an external ventricular drain (EVD) may be placed to monitor and control ICP. This also permits calculation of the CPP

- *Blood*: treatment options depend on the sort of bleed and clinical context. An EDH requires immediate neurosurgical evacuation via a trauma craniotomy before ICP exponentially rises to cause brainstem tonsillar herniation. A chronic SDH requires Burr hole evacuation and drainage. The management for aneurysmal subarachnoid bleeds either requires emergency coiling, placement of an EVD to treat acute hydrocephalus or craniotomy and clipping
- *Brain*: if a tumour is the underlying diagnosis, the management before definitive surgery to debulk the lesion requires treating the signs and symptoms, e.g. steroids, PPIs, laxatives.

Depending on the disease process, the patient may require intubation and ventilation to help control $PaCO_2$, and hence ICP, e.g. if PaO_2 is >12 kPa, $PaCO_2$ <6 kPa and FiO_2 is 0.4, then the patient may not require intubation. Other than controlling the ventilation, MAP might be maintained >90mmHg to help maintain CPP >65 mmHg.

Hyponatraemia may occur due to over-hydration, the stress response with sodium and water retention or the syndrome of inappropriate ADH (SIADH). This has to be managed by careful fluid and electrolyte balance, since hyponatraemia may lead to further neurological impairment and cerebral oedema.

Spinal injury

What are the patterns of deficit seen in some spinal cord syndromes?

The emergency management of spinal cord injury is according to the ATLS$^{®}$ protocol, but some syndromes can develop in critically ill patients due to other co-existing morbidities

- *Central cord syndrome*: damage to the central canal and innermost aspects of the spinal cord produces motor weakness, mainly affecting the upper limbs. Sensory loss is usually less severe
- *Anterior spinal cord syndrome*: this is due to damage of the anterior aspect of the spinal cord, resulting in loss of motor function. There is also loss of pain and temperature sensation, but light touch, proprioception and vibration sense are unaffected owing to preservation of the dorsal columns
- *Brown–Séquard syndrome*: occurs from hemisection of the spinal cord causing motor loss below the lesion, and contralateral loss of pain and temperature sensation. There is ipsilateral loss of dorsal column function

What deficits are seen in cases of complete injury?

The following deficits can occur

- *Motor deficit*: an initial flaccid paralysis below the level of the lesion gives way to a spastic paralysis with increased tone and deep tendon reflexes due to loss of upper motor neurone input into the cord

- *Sensory deficit*: this affects the anterolateral and posterior columns, affecting the somatic and visceral components to sensation
- *Autonomic deficit*: affecting the sympathetic and parasympathetic outputs of the cord, e.g. hyperhidrosis

Why may trauma to the spinal injury result in bradycardia?

The following process may produce a bradycardia from trauma of any cause

- *Sympathetic*: the sympathetic outflow is lost from the damaged cord
- *Parasympathetic*: a reflex increase in the cranial parasympathetic outflow can occur due to airway suctioning
- *Cushing reflex*: due to elevated intracranial pressure if there is an associated head injury
- *Co-morbidities*: due to cardiac disease or the use of drugs, e.g. β-adrenoceptor blockers

Why may spinal cord lesions lead to hypotension?

The spinal cord-induced bradycardia and drop in cardiac output can be exacerbated by hypotension due to

- *Sympathetic*: loss of sympathetic outflow eliminates vasomotor tone leading to reduced systemic vascular resistance and, therefore, reduced arterial pressure. If combined to the bradycardia, the cardiac output drops further reducing the arterial pressure

- *Occult blood loss*: e.g. following blunt abdominal trauma. Haemorrhage may be missed as it is easy to ascribe hypotension to the spinal injury alone

What are the dangers of autonomic dysfunction in these situations?

Occult blood loss may be missed if there is hypotension erroneously ascribed to spinal trauma. This may lead to

- *Volume overload*: over-hydration can occur during fluid resuscitation, leading to pulmonary oedema
- *Reduced cerebral perfusion pressure (CPP)*: hypotension reduces the CPP in the face of a head injury and rising intracranial pressure
- *Hypothermia*: this may be caused due to loss of vasomotor control

Bradycardia may be exacerbated when carrying out manoeuvres that stimulate the cranial parasympathetic outflow, e.g. intubation, airway suction, bladder distension. This may induce cardiac arrest; therefore, IV atropine should be at hand to reverse this process.

What is 'spinal shock'?

This is a temporary state of flaccid paralysis that usually occurs very soon after a spinal injury, and may take 3–4 weeks to resolve. This is due to the loss of excitatory stimuli from supraspinal levels.

What drug has been used to minimise the extent of spinal injury following trauma?

High-dose IV methylprednisolone has been used to limit secondary spinal injury from free radicals produced following trauma. For the most beneficial effect, it must be given within 8 hours of trauma, but check with your local regional spinal injuries centre as this has become controversial.

What are the important issues surrounding long-term management?

The most important aspect of long-term management is rehabilitation. Prevention of decubitus ulcers from immobilisation is a priority. Nutritional support for high spinal injuries in the form of percutaneous enteral feeding, e.g. a Hickman line, is needed to meet the increased metabolic demands and risk of aspiration due to lying supine. Bowel care, with regular enemas and bulk-forming agents, bladder care, with intermittent catheterisation, and physiotherapy to help clear lung secretions and prevent limb contractures, form the basics. A mini tracheostomy may be required, and psychological support and counselling are strongly encouraged.

Procedures

Lumbar puncture

What is the purpose of a lumbar puncture (LP)?

There are multiple reasons to conduct an LP to siphon CSF from the subarachnoid space, but some of the most common indications include

- Infection, e.g. meningitis, encephalitis
- Blood, e.g. subarachnoid haemorrhage
- Hydrocephalus, e.g. therapeutic management and high opening pressures might be present

The majority are inserted on the ward under direct vision and CSF is sent for visual, microbiological, cytological and biochemical analysis. It requires some basic expertise and some pre-procedure checks

What are the pre-procedure checks required for a safe insertion?

An LP should be conducted on the basis of necessity and time, e.g. the timing following an SAH is crucial (12 h post-ictus), and a full ABCDE assessment should be performed. Some common checks include

- Laboratory
  - *Prothrombin time (PT)*: e.g. in patients on warfarin anticoagulation, as this can cause a devastating haematoma to form in any one of the potential meningeal spaces in the spine
  - *Platelet count*: in patients at risk of prolonged bleeding due to haematological diseases, e.g. haemophilia, it is prudent to check
- Radiological
  - *CT*: this is mandatory if there is a clinical suspicion of a space, occupying lesion, e.g. tumour, due to the clinical history (reduced GCS, seizure or focal neurological signs), as it can cause devastating cerebral herniation, and in the

case of an SAH, it should only be carried out 12 hours
post-ictus. Suspected raised ICP is also a contraindication

- Microbiology
  - *Sepsis*: the presence of infection overlying the insertion
    site is an absolute contraindication due to the risk of
    meningitis, encephalitis, and spinal and cranial abscess
    formation

Written informed consent from the patient should be obtained
to both the LP and appropriate local anaesthetic (and light
sedation if necessary). This procedure can be carried out on
the ward (i.e. Level 0) but patients should be closely monitored
to detect potential complications.

List the equipment needed and outline the steps for insertion?

An assembly of equipment is needed and includes a sterile
pack, drapes, gauze swabs, selection of needles, sterile gloves,
antiseptic solution, local anaesthetic, LP needle, manometer,
up to four universal containers and dressings, all opened in an
aseptic non-touch sterile technique.

- *Positioning*: the patient is positioned on their side and their
  legs are drawn up into a foetal position
- *Marking*: the surface marking of the top of the iliac crests
  concurs to the termination of the spinal cord, e.g. L3–4
- *Prep and drape*: the skin needs to be thoroughly cleaned
  using Betadine® and the patient draped in an aseptic
  non-touch sterile technique

- *Infiltration of local anaesthetic (LA)*: e.g. 2 ml 2% lignocaine (lidocaine) is used to make a small wheal over the skin using an orange needle before 5–10 ml is used to progressively infiltrate the subcutaneous layers surrounding the vertebral column using a green needle
- *Insertion of LP needle*: the needle is passed with the eye (cutting point) facing upwards. The needle is passed through the space between the spinous processes at the corresponding level until a slight give is felt
- *Manometry*: once CSF is seen inside the LP needle it is withdrawn, but the cannula is left in place and manometer is attached to measure the opening pressure ($\sim$5–20 cmH$_2$O)
- *Collection*: up to four universal containers are used to siphon off CSF once the opening pressure is measured, and routine tests include virology, cytology, protein and glucose, and culture. Only 3–5 ml needs to be placed in each bottle

The CSF is inspected for its general appearance and analysed for its protein (0.18–0.45) and glucose content (2.5–3.5 mmol/L), glucose CSF: serum ratio (normally 0.6) and white cell count (normally <3). Following successful collection of CSF, the patient is kept supine for several hours and observed for potential complications.

What are the complications of LP insertion?
The complications include

- Minor
  - Headache
  - Lumbar tenderness

- ■ Limb parasthesiae
- Late
  - ■ Haematoma, e.g. epidural
  - ■ Infection, e.g. arachnoiditis
  - ■ Paraplegia

Bibliography

American College of Surgeons. Head trauma. In *Advanced Trauma Life Support*® *(ATLS*®*)*, 9th edn. Chicago, IL, American College of Surgeons; 2012: Chapter 7.

Liebenberg WA, Johnson RD. *Neurosurgery for Basic Surgical Trainees*, 2nd edn. Carnforth, Hippocrates Books; 2010.

Chapter 5

Exposure (everything else)

Renal

Acid–base balance

Define the pH

pH is $-\log^{10} [H^+]$.

What is the pH of blood?

7.35–7.45.

Where does the acid load (H^+) in the body come from?

Most of the H^+ in the body comes from CO_2 generated from metabolism. This enters solution, forming carbonic acid through a reaction mediated by the enzyme carbonic anhydrase

$$CO_2 + H_2O = H_2CO_3 = H^+ + HCO_3^-$$

Acid is also generated by

- Metabolism
  - Of sulphur-containing amino acids, cysteine and methionine
  - Generation of lactic acid during anaerobic metabolism

- Generating the ketone bodies acetone, acetoacetate and β-hydroxybutyrate, e.g. diabetic ketoacidosis (DKA)

What are the main buffer systems in the intravascular, interstitial and intracellular compartments?

In the plasma the main systems are

- Bicarbonate (HCO_3^-)
- Phosphate (PO_4^{3-})
- Plasma proteins
- Globin component of haemoglobin

The bicarbonate system is predominantly interstitial, and cytoplasmic proteins are mostly intracellular

What does the Henderson–Hasselbalch equation describe?

This defines the relationship between dissociated and undissociated acids and bases

$$CO_2 + H_2O = H_2CO_3 = H^+ + HCO_3^-$$

$$pH = 6.1 + \log \frac{[HCO_3^-]}{pCO_2 \times 0.23}.$$

Which organ systems are involved in regulating acid–base balance?

- *Respiratory system*: this controls $PaCO_2$ through alterations in alveolar ventilation. CO_2 indirectly stimulates central chemoreceptors (in the medulla oblongata) by releasing H^+, which once it crosses the blood–brain barrier (BBB), dissolves in the cerebrospinal fluid (CSF)

- *Renal*: this controls the $[HCO_3^-]$ and is important for long-term control and compensation of acid–base disturbances
- *Haematology*: the constituents of blood, e.g. plasma proteins and haemoglobin, serve as buffers
- *Rheumatology*: H^+ may exchange with cations from bone mineral. Also, carbonate in bone can be used to support plasma HCO_3^- levels
- *Gastrointestinal*: the liver may generate HCO_3^- and NH_4^+ (ammonium) by glutamine metabolism. In the kidney tubules, ammonia excretion generates more bicarbonate

How does the kidney absorb bicarbonate?

There are three main methods by which the kidneys increase the plasma bicarbonate

- Replacement
    - *Tubule cells*: can replace filtered bicarbonate and phosphate with bicarbonate that is generated in the tubular cells
- Generation
    - *Tubule cells*: can generate *de novo* bicarbonate from glutamine that is absorbed by tubule cells

Define the base deficit (base excess)?

The base deficit is the amount of acid or alkali required to restore 1 L of fully oxygenated blood to a normal pH at a pCO_2

of 5.3 kPa at 37°C. It helps to indicate if an acid–base disturbance is respiratory, metabolic or mixed, and usually ranges from −2 to +2 mmol/L.

What basic investigation provides information on acid–base balance?

This is the arterial blood gas (ABG), which is usually taken from venepuncture of the radial artery. It provides basic information, including pH, $PaCO_2$ (4.5–6.0 kPa), HCO_3^- (22–28 mmol/L), PaO_2 (10.5–13.5 kPa) and base excess. It should be interpreted in that order (*see* below). Other valuable information is lactate, indicating inadequate tissue perfusion (0–2 mmol/L) and glucose, as a guide to treatment in diabetic ketoacidosis.

How is knowledge of the PaO_2 useful?

It provides a guide to tissue oxygenation, but should be interpreted compared to the FiO_2. A relatively normal PaO_2 but a high FiO_2 can indicate problems diffusing oxygen from the alveolus into blood, e.g. inefficient gas exchange.

Describe some common acid–base disturbances on ABG analysis?

The pH influences the analysis of other variables if it is respiratory, metabolic, or mixed.

pH

- Acidosis (<7.35)
  - *Respiratory*: raised $PaCO_2$ and normal/raised HCO_3^- (if metabolic compensation)

- *Metabolic*: normal/low $PaCO_2$ (if respiratory compensation) and low HCO_3^-
  - Alkalosis (>7.45)
    - *Respiratory*: low $PaCO_2$ and normal/low HCO_3^- (if metabolic compensation)
    - *Metabolic*: normal/raised $PaCO_2$ (if respiratory compensation) and raised HCO_3^-

Metabolic acidosis

What is metabolic acidosis?

This is an acid–base disturbance characterised by an increase in the total body acid (pH <7.35). There is also a fall of the serum bicarbonate to below the reference range.

In what ways may bicarbonate be lost in the cases of metabolic acidosis?

The bicarbonate may be

- Excreted, e.g. vomiting, diarrhoea, fistulas or urine
- Depleted through buffering an overwhelming H^+ load
- Impaired generation of bicarbonate

How may the causes of metabolic acidosis be classified?

The causes may be classified according to the anion gap

$$\text{Anion gap} = (Na^+ + K^+) - (HCO_3^- + Cl^-)$$

The anion gap ranges from ~ 12 to 20 mmol/L and estimates the contribution of unmeasured ions, e.g. lactate, to help determine the cause of a metabolic acidosis.

- Normal anion gap due to loss of bicarbonate (or ingestion of acid)
  - *Gastrointestinal*: this includes diarrhoea, pancreatic fistula, ileostomy and ingestion of acidifying agents, e.g. TPN and excess amino acids
  - *Renal*: losses of bicarbonate include renal failure, and tubular acidosis Type II and Type IV (hypoaldosteronism)

Chloride ions replace bicarbonate to ensure electrochemical neutrality, but can lead to a hyperchloraemia

- Increased anion gap (increased exogenous or endogenous acid ingestion)
  - *K*etoacidosis, e.g. DKA, starvation, alcoholism
  - *U*raemia
  - *S*alicylate poisoning
  - *M*ethanol intoxication
  - *(A)*ethylene glycol poisoning
  - *L*actic acidosis, e.g. sepsis, shock, hypermetabolic state such as burns

The acronym **KUSsMAuL** is useful, particularly as Kussmaul's respiration is a clinical sign of metabolic acidosis. Bicarbonate buffers the acid load. It is catalysed to CO_2, and H_2O, which is then excreted by the lungs.

What effects can acidosis have on body physiology?
- Shift of the oxygen dissociation curve to the right, signifying a reduction of the haemoglobin molecule's oxygen affinity. This increases tissue oxygenation

- Decreased myocardial contractility
- Resistance to the effects of circulating catecholamines
- Pulmonary hypertension, as acidosis causes pulmonary vasoconstriction
- Cardiac arrhythmias, due to both a direct effect and through development of hyperkalaemia
- Increased sympathetic activity and paradoxical catecholamine resistance

What are the principles of management of any cause of metabolic acidosis?

The principles of management involve

- *Assessment*: of the severity of the acidosis and resultant complications mentioned above
- *Management*: of the underlying cause, e.g. fluids and insulin for DKA, emergency dialysis for renal failure

The use of bicarbonate is a controversial issue. It is more justified in cases of hyperchloraemic metabolic acidosis, where the primary problem is a loss of bicarbonate (*see* Lactic Acidosis), but renal involvement is important.

Metabolic alkalosis

What is the essential disturbance that defines a metabolic alkalosis?

The essential change is a primary increase in the serum bicarbonate to >28 mmol/L.

Which ions other than bicarbonate are implicated in the development of metabolic alkalosis?

The other ions are

- *Hydrogen ions (protons)*: loss of protons, e.g. by vomiting, leads to a compensatory increase in bicarbonate and, hence, alkalosis
- *Chloride ions*: loss causes renal tubules to increase bicarbonate uptake in order to maintain electrochemical neutrality, as the loss of one leads to gain of the other
- *Potassium*: loss of this ion leads to increased absorption of bicarbonate in the renal tubules. Also, this leads to increased cellular uptake of protons

Which organ system is most commonly involved in metabolic alkalosis?

Gut pathology is often implicated.

Give some examples of the causes of metabolic alkalosis

- Excess bicarbonate ingestion
  - *Gastrointestinal*: e.g. milk–alkali syndrome
  - *Iatrogenic*: overtreatment of acidosis
- Inappropriate acid loss (with gain of bicarbonate)
  - *Gastrointestinal*: persistent vomiting, e.g. pyloric stenosis, self-induced vomiting
  - *Metabolic*: any cause of hypokalaemia, as this shifts protons into cells
  - *Endocrine*: hyperaldosteronism
  - *Iatrogenic*: chloride loss, e.g. secondary to diuretic abuse

One other cause is contraction alkalosis due to rapid diuresis or fulminant liver failure. This increases bicarbonate absorption over chloride.

Describe the mechanism by which metabolic alkalosis develops in cases of pyloric stenosis

In the case of pyloric stenosis, metabolic alkalosis develops and is perpetuated by normal compensatory mechanisms

- Gastric acid is a rich source of protons and chloride, which are both lost in vomit
- There is a reduction of pancreatic juice secretion due to reduced acid load at the duodenum, which therefore retains bicarbonate
- Volume depletion maintains the alkalosis by leading to bicarbonate absorption over chloride, e.g. contraction alkalosis
- There is increased uptake of bicarbonate at renal tubules (response to a loss of chloride) in order to maintain electrochemical neutrality

Why may patients with a metabolic alkalosis develop poor tissue oxygenation?

There are two main reasons

- As part of the body's compensatory response to alkalosis, there is hypoventilation in order to increase the $PaCO_2$
- Alkalosis causes a shift of the oxygen dissociation curve to the left, signifying increased haemoglobin affinity for oxygen, at the expense of tissue oxygen uptake

Lactic acidosis

What are the defining features of lactic acidosis?

The important features include a metabolic acidosis (with varying degrees of compensation) and elevated serum lactate. The serum lactate level is normally <2 mmol/L, but with lactic acidosis, it may increase to >5 mmol/L.

How may the causes of lactic acidosis be classified?

The Cohen and Woods (1976) classification divides the causes thus

- Type A: clinical evidence of inadequate tissue oxygenation
  - *Anaerobic metabolism*: e.g. sprinting, marathon running, seizures and lactate is produced from pyruvate
  - *Shock (any cause)*: causing poor tissue perfusion and cellular hypoxia, worsening the anaerobic metabolism, e.g. mesenteric ischaemia, haemorrhagic shock
  - *Reduced tissue oxygenation*: tissue perfusion may be adequate but oxygen delivery and utilisation may be inadequate, e.g. carbon monoxide poisoning, extremely severe anaemia
- Type B: no clinical evidence of inadequate tissue oxygenation
  - *Type B1 (chronic diseases)*: including liver disease, renal failure, DKA, malignancy, short bowel syndrome
  - *Type B2 (drug-induced)*: including paracetamol, salicylate overdose, metformin, adrenaline, alcohol intoxication, anti-retroviral medication

- *Type B3 (metabolism)*: inborn errors, e.g. congenital forms of lactic acidosis due to pyruvate dehydrogenase deficiency

What are the essential findings on investigation?

The diagnostic features are an elevated serum lactate and the presence of an increased anion gap metabolic acidosis on ABG analysis in the face of known predisposing factors.

What are the principles of management of lactic acidosis?

The most important aspect of management is

- Correcting the predisposing factor, e.g. support of the cardiac output in order to improve the tissue perfusion

What are the precautions and potential problems associated with bicarbonate therapy?

Some considerations must be made when using bicarbonate to reverse metabolic acidosis

- *Rate*: bicarbonate must be infused slowly. It comes as a hypertonic 8.4% solution (or hypotonic 1.26% solution), which can alter myocardial contractility depending on the rate of infusion
- *Dose*: it must be carefully titrated to the desired therapeutic end point, because of the risk of an overshoot metabolic acidosis

Complications can include

- *Overshoot alkalosis*: this shifts the oxygen dissociation curve to the left, reducing oxygen delivery to the tissues
- *Respiratory acidosis*: extra CO_2 is generated upon the use of bicarbonate to mop up excess protons. If ventilation is inadequate, respiratory acidosis may develop
- *Intracellular acidosis*: may also be worsened by the use of bicarbonate, as CO_2 rapidly diffuses across cell membranes. This CO_2 then dissolves in the cytoplasm (*and* CSF) generating extra protons, worsening intracellular, and intracerebral, acidosis

Electrolyte balance: calcium (and phosphate)

What is the normal level of serum calcium?
2.2–2.6 mmol/L.

What is the distribution of calcium in the body?
Ninety-nine per cent of calcium is found in bone, mostly as hydroxyapatite. One per cent is readily exchangeable as calcium phosphate salts.

In what state is calcium found in the circulation?
- 50% is unbound and ionised
- 45% is bound to plasma proteins
- 5% is associated with anions such as citrate and lactate

Which organ systems are involved in controlling serum calcium levels?
The main organ systems include the gut, kidneys and skeletal systems.

Name the hormones involved in controlling serum calcium

Major hormones

- *Parathyroid hormone (PTH)*: an 84-amino acid molecule, produced by the parathyroid glands
- *Vitamin D_3 (cholecalciferol) metabolites*: this is obtained from the diet and the skin
- *Calcitonin*: a 32-amino acid molecule, produced by parafollicular (C) cells in the thyroid gland

Other hormones include parathyroid hormone-related peptide (PTHrP), and magnesium and albumin also play a role. Magnesium prevents PTH release, potentially causing hypocalcaemia. Up to 40% of plasma calcium is bound to albumin. It is important that the unbound ionised form is measured, e.g. add 0.1 mmol/L to the level for every 4 g/L drop in albumin $<$40 g/L.

Briefly describe their effects

- PTH (raised Ca^{2+} but low PO_4^{3-})
  - *Bone*: increases the synthesis of enzymes that break down bone matrix to release calcium and phosphate into the circulation. It also stimulates osteocytic and osteoclastic activity, leading to progressive bone reabsorption
  - *Renal*: increases renal phosphate excretion while reducing renal calcium loss. It also stimulates 1-α-hydroxylase activity in the kidney, increasing 1,25 dihydroxy-vitamin D_3 (calcitriol), thus indirectly increasing calcium absorption

- Vitamin D_3 (cholecalciferol) metabolites ($\uparrow Ca^{2+}$ and $\uparrow PO_4^{3-}$ but $\downarrow$PTH release)
  - *Bone*: calcitriol increases both serum calcium and the calcification of bone matrix. It stimulates osteoblastic proliferation and protein synthesis
  - *Renal*: it promotes calcium and phosphate reabsorption
  - *Gastrointestinal*: it enhances gut absorption of calcium and phosphate
- Calcitonin ($\downarrow Ca^{2+}$ and $\downarrow PO_4^{3-}$)
  - *Bone*: inhibits bone resorption through inhibition of osteoclastic activity if serum calcium >2.6 mmol/L
  - *Renal*: stimulates the excretion of sodium, chloride, calcium and phosphate

What are the clinical consequences of hypercalcaemia?

- *Renal*: calculi due to hypercalcinuria, nephrocalcinosis and multi-focal calcium deposits in the renal parenchyma. Polyuria and polydipsia occur due to decreased tubular function. This can lead to dehydration, especially if there is associated vomiting
- *Gastrointestinal*: dyspepsia and peptic ulceration due to increased gastric acid secretion stimulated by calcium and PTH. There is an increased risk of developing acute pancreatitis, and constipation is common
- *Bone*: cysts can develop, osteitis fibrosa cystica and Brown's tumours may occur
- *General medical*: a non-specific series of symptoms can develop, e.g. tiredness, lethargy and organic psychosis, and, in severe cases, this can lead to coma

What ECG changes may be found?

The ECG changes are related to alterations in the membrane potential and cardiac conduction, and include

- Shortened QT interval
- Increased PR interval (progressing to heart block)
- Flattened or inverted T-waves

Under what circumstances may a surgeon encounter a patient with hypercalcaemia?

The main reasons why a surgeon may encounter a hypercalcaemic patient are

- *Malignancy*: a hypercalcaemia of malignancy may develop, e.g. bronchogenic carcinoma and pathological fractures due to secondary deposits
- *Endocrine*: primary hyperparathyroidism, due to an adenoma of the parathyroid gland, requiring neck exploration, and tertiary hyperparathyroidism in renal transplant patients
- *General complications*: urinary obstruction due to renal calculi, deranged physiology from acute pancreatitis and peptic ulceration

What are the differential diagnoses of abdominal pain in the hypercalcaemic patient?

- Peptic ulceration (perforation may be present)
- Renal colic from calculi
- Acute pancreatitis
- Constipation from reduced intestinal motility

What does the emergency management of hypercalcaemia involve?

Management of acute hypercalcaemia (>3.5 mmol/L), following immediate ABCDE assessment, involves

- Commencing continuous cardiac monitoring
- Fluid resuscitation by giving 3000 ml of normal saline in 24 hours. To prevent overload, CVP monitoring may be required. Furosemide can be given to help aid calcium diuresis and prevent overload
- Urinary catheter to monitor fluid balance and urinary volumes, e.g. output should be >2000 ml/day
- A bisphosphonate infusion can rapidly reduce the serum calcium, e.g. pamidronate, but should only be given once fully rehydrated
- High-dose steroids, e.g. 40 mg of prednisolone, is useful in some cases, such as myeloma, sarcoidosis or haematological malignancies

In all cases, identifying and treating the underlying cause by conducting basic laboratory investigations, e.g. PTH, is required. Surgery is required in those cases due to hyperparathyroidism.

What is the most important surgical cause of hypocalcaemia?

The most important surgical cause is after thyroid surgery, when there is inadvertent removal of the parathyroid glands.

Give some of the recognised features of hypocalcaemia?

The important clinical features are

- *Neurological*: irritability manifest as peripheral and circumoral parathesiae
- *Muscular*: cramps
- *Tetany*: spasms
- *Chvostek's sign*: twitching of the facial muscles on tapping of the facial nerve anterior to the tragus
- *Trousseau's sign*: tetanic spasm of the hand upon tapping the median nerve following blood pressure cuff-induced arm ischaemia

What is the emergency management of hypocalcaemia?
- Commencement of cardiac monitoring
- Fluid resuscitation
- Give 10 ml of 10% calcium gluconate IV, followed by 10–40 ml in a saline infusion over 4–8 hours

Consider treating hypomagnesaemia if present and getting cardiology advice if digitalis toxicity is present, as rapid correction might lead to cardiac arrest.

Electrolyte balance: magnesium

What is the normal serum level of magnesium?
0.7–1.0 mmol/L.

What is the distribution of magnesium in the body?
Magnesium is the second most abundant intracellular cation after potassium. The total body magnesium is ~25 g. Up to 65% is located in bone and only 1% is found in serum. Therefore, serum is a poor reflection of the total body store.

What purpose does magnesium serve?

Magnesium is an essential co-factor in a number of enzymes, notably in the transfer of phosphate groups, and protein synthesis. It is most conspicuously important for the normal function of the central nervous system, neuromuscular and cardiovascular systems.

What is the relationship between magnesium and serum calcium?

High magnesium levels prevent calcium cellular uptake, and for this reason hypermagnesaemia can lead to bradycardia and sluggish deep tendon reflexes.

What drug is used to reverse the effects of severe hypermagnesaemia?

Calcium gluconate.

Which organ is largely responsible for magnesium homeostasis?

The kidney is the major site for magnesium balance. It is freely filtered at the glomerulus, and reabsorbed mainly at the proximal convoluted tubule and the thick ascending limb of the loop of Henle.

What are the main causes of hypomagnesaemia?

- Decreased intake
  - *Starvation*: e.g. alcoholism, malnutrition
- Increased excretion

- *Gastrointestinal losses*: e.g. diarrhoea, inflammatory bowel disease, intestinal resection and bypasses
- *Renal*: any state of diuresis, e.g. diuretic use, diuretic phase of acute renal failure, hypercalcaemia
- *Endocrine*: e.g. diabetes mellitus, hyperparathyroidism, hyperthyroidism

How common is hypomagnesaemia in the hospital setting?
Hypomagnesaemia occurs in over 60% of the critically ill, most commonly associated with diuretic use.

How can hypomagnesaemia be recognised?
It may be difficult to recognise hypomagnesaemia due to its varied presentation. Recognised features include

- Arrhythmias, e.g. AF
- ECG changes, e.g. a prolonged PR interval ($>$220 ms) and widened QRS complexes
- Muscular weakness
- Confusion

Give some examples of the therapeutic role of magnesium-containing compounds
- *Anti-arrhythmic*: can be used to achieve chemical cardioversion for acute AF
- *Acute MI*: some studies suggest a survival benefit from early administration
- *Antacid*: e.g. magnesium trisilicate, or hydroxide
- *Laxative*: e.g. magnesium sulphate

- *Eclampsia*: for the prevention of recurrent seizures in this condition
- *Acute asthma*: it has a role to play in both acute asthma and COPD

Electrolyte balance: potassium

What is the normal level of serum potassium?

3.5–5.0 mmol/L.

What is the distribution of potassium in the body?

Ninety-eight per cent of potassium is intracellular at a concentration of ~150 mmol/L, compared to ~4 mmol/L in the serum.

How is potassium regulated?

There are a number of influential factors on serum potassium

- Gastrointestinal
  - *Diet*: the Western diet may contain 20–100 mmol of potassium daily
- Endocrine
  - *Aldosterone*: this mineralocorticoid, produced by the zona glomerulosa of the adrenal gland, stimulates sodium reabsorption in the distal convoluted tubule and cortical collecting duct, through an active exchange with potassium. It promotes its excretion
  - *Insulin*: stimulates potassium uptake into cells, reducing the serum level

- Renal
  - *Acid–base balance*: potassium and H^+ are exchanged at the cell membrane, producing reciprocal changes in concentration, e.g. acidosis leads to hyperkalaemia. Similarly, alkalosis can lead to hypokalaemia. Also, renal reabsorption of one causes excretion of the other
  - *Tubular fluid flow rate*: increased flow promotes potassium secretion, one method by which diuretics may cause hypokalaemia

What are the causes of hyperkalaemia?
- Artefact, e.g. haemolysis in the blood bottle
- Excess administration, e.g. IV fluids
- Redistribution
  - *Compartmental fluid shifts*: due to injury, intravascular haemolysis, burns, rhabdomyolysis, tissue necrosis, massive blood transfusion
  - *Reduced cellular uptake*: e.g. insulin deficiency, acidosis
- Decreased excretion
  - *Renal*: e.g. renal failure, potassium-sparing diuretics
  - *Endocrine*: e.g. Addison's disease, mineralocorticoid resistance due to systemic lupus erythematosus (SLE)

What ECG changes may be found in hyper- and hypokalaemia?
- Hyperkalaemia
  - Tall tented T-waves
  - Small P-waves
  - Widened QRS complexes

- Ventricular fibrillation (there is no pulse at this stage)
- Hypokalaemia
  - Small or inverted T-waves
  - Prominent U-waves (seen after T-waves)
  - Prolonged PR interval
  - ST segment depression

What is the emergency management of hyperkalaemia?

The serum potassium must be re-checked to determine if it is a spurious finding. If it comes back as >6.5 mmol/L, following immediate ABCDE assessment, implement

- Continuous cardiac monitoring
- Stop all potassium-containing intravenous fluids, including Hartmann's
- Calcium gluconate (10 ml of 10%) is given IV over 10 min, which provides a short-term cardioprotective effect but does not decease the serum potassium
- Give 5–10 U of insulin in 50 ml of 50% dextrose IV over 30 minutes, which increases cellular uptake of potassium
- Calcium resonium (15 g PO or 30 g PR) can be given to provide longer term potassium depletion

In all cases, treat the underlying cause and investigate renal function, as haemodialysis might be needed if the potassium is persistently high or if there is severe acidosis (pH <7.20). The use of bicarbonate is a specialist renal intervention as it can paradoxically exacerbate the acidosis.

What use does knowledge of the cardiac effects of potassium have for surgical practice?

Potassium-rich cardioplegic solutions are used to arrest the heart in diastole to permit cardiac surgery once cardiopulmonary bypass has been established.

What are the causes of hypokalaemia?

- Artefact, e.g. drip arm sampling
- Decreased intake
  - *Starvation*: e.g. alcoholism
- Redistribution
  - *Compartmental fluid shifts*: including alkalosis and insulin excess
- Increased excretion
  - *Gastrointestinal losses*: e.g. vomiting and diarrhoea, enterocutaneous fistula, mucin-secreting adenomas of the colon
  - *Renal losses*: e.g. diuretics including loop and thiazides, renal tubular acidosis
  - *Endocrine*: e.g. Conn's and Cushing's syndromes

It is difficult to correct hypokalaemia if co-existing hypomagnesaemia is present.

What are the clinical features associated with hypokalaemia?

- Muscular weakness and cramps
- Lethargy and confusion
- Atrial and ventricular arrhythmias

- Increased digoxin toxicity
- Paralytic ileus

Electrolyte balance: sodium

What is the normal level of serum sodium?
135–145 mmol/L.

What is the distribution of sodium in the body?
Sodium is the major extracellular cation in the body

- 50% is extracellular
- 45% is in bone
- 5% is intracellular

The vast majority (~70%) is found in the readily exchangeable form.

What are the major physiological roles of sodium?
It exerts significant osmotic forces, and is important for maintaining water balance between intracellular and extracellular compartments. This contributes to external water balance and extracellular fluid volume. It is important in generating action potentials.

What is the daily sodium requirement?
The daily requirement is about 1 mmol/kg/day.

Give a simple classification of the causes of hyponatraemia?
- Water excess
  - *Increased uptake (oedematous)*: polydipsia, iatrogenic, e.g. TURP syndrome, excess dextrose administration

- Retention of water (oedematous): SIADH
- *Retention of water and salt*: nephrotic syndrome, cardiac, hepatic and renal failure
- Water loss (sodium loss is in excess)
  - *Renal losses (urinary sodium >20 mmol/L)*: diuretic excess, diuretic phase of renal failure, Addison's disease, relief of chronic urinary obstruction, osmolar diuresis, e.g. glucose
  - *Non-renal losses (urinary sodium <20 mmol/L)*: gut losses, e.g. diarrhoea, vomiting, fistulas, small bowel obstruction and trauma, e.g. burns

What is pseudohyponatraemia?

This is a falsely low sodium concentration due to an increased serum volume secondary to hyperlipidaemia or hyperproteinaemia.

What is the TURP syndrome?

This is a syndrome of cardiovascular and neurological symptoms, occurring after the use of irrigation fluid containing hypotonic glycine during transurethral resection of the prostate (TURP). The fluid is absorbed through injured vessels, producing a dilutional hyponatraemia. It leads to haemodynamic instability, confusion and in severe cases, convulsions and coma.

Which disease processes may trigger the syndrome of inappropriate ADH secretion (SIADH)?

SIADH may be triggered by the following

- Lung pathology
  - Infection, e.g. pneumonia, aspergillosis, abscess, TB
- Malignancy
  - Small cell lung carcinoma
  - Brain tumours
  - Prostatic carcinoma
- Intracranial pathology
  - Infection, e.g. meningitis, abscess, Guillain-Barré syndrome
  - Head injury
  - Haemorrhage, e.g. subarachnoid, subdural
  - Surgery, e.g. pituitary

Other causes include alcohol withdrawal, trauma, opiates and symptomatic HIV.

What does the term 'inappropriate' refer to in SIADH?

There is a pathological retention of water in the absence of renal, adrenal or thyroid disease, and urine osmolality is inappropriately high in relation to the plasma osmolality.

What are clinical features of hyponatraemia?

The symptoms are due to fluid overload in neurons, and include confusion, agitation, fits and reduced GCS. Other features depend on the underlying cause, and the most appropriate management is to treat the underlying cause.

What are the causes of hypernatraemia?

The major causes may be classified as

- Water loss (in excess of sodium)
  - Fluid loss (but no water replacement), e.g. vomiting, diarrhoea, burns
  - Incorrect fluid replacement, e.g. excess saline
  - Diabetes insipidus
  - Osmotic diuresis, e.g. hyperglycaemia
  - Primary hyperaldosteronism
- Sodium excess (in excess of water)
  - Incorrect fluid replacement, e.g. excess saline
  - Primary hyperaldosteronism

What is diabetes insipidus?

This is polyuria producing hypovolaemia and a resultant hypernatraemia with dehydration, due to either a renal insensitivity to (nephrogenic) or deficiency of (cranial). The inability to concentrate urine results in a polydipsia to compensate for the excess urinary losses.

Oliguria: low urine output state

What is the purpose of measuring the urine output in the post-operative patient?

Since the urine output is determined by the renal perfusion pressure, measurement provides a useful index of the cardiac output, and the ability to adequately oxygenate the peripheral tissues. It is also an indicator of renal tubular function, independent of the renal perfusion and cardiac output.

What is the minimum acceptable urine output in adults and children?

In adults, the minimum acceptable urine output is 0.5 ml/kg/h and in children it is 1 ml/kg/h.

What factors determine the urine output?

- Adequate renal perfusion pressure, determined by the cardiac output and the arteriolar tone
- Normal renal tubular function
- Patent urinary tract distal to the kidneys

What are the common causes of post-operative oliguria?

- Physiological stress response
- Poor renal perfusion
  - Dehydration (underfilling)
  - Bleeding
  - Low cardiac output state
  - Vasodilatation, e.g. due to septic shock
- Renal tubular dysfunction, e.g. acute tubular necrosis and established renal failure
- Renal tract obstruction, e.g. due to stones, extrinsic compression, blocked urinary catheter
- Intra-abdominal hypertension (>20 mmHg) can occur secondary to bowel obstruction, retroperitoneal collection (causing compression of the renal parenchyma)

Which pathologies may lead to a post-operative low cardiac output state?

A low cardiac output state post-operatively may be caused by

- Myocardial infarction and pulmonary embolism in the post-operative period, e.g. following hip surgery
- Myocardial arrhythmias, e.g. fast AF and VT
- Requirement for positive pressure ventilation, which reduces venous return (to the right side of the heart)
- Excess fluid administration, leading to cardiac failure in those with poor ventricular function

What is the most common and benign reason for post-operative oliguria?

The most common cause is due to the physiological stress response to surgery in the first 24–36 hours post-operatively. This is due to circulating glucocorticoids and mineralocorticoids inducing salt and water retention. Trauma and various anaesthetic gases also stimulate the release of vasopressin from the posterior pituitary, stimulating post-operative solute-free water retention.

What signs would you look for when examining a post-operative patient with a low urine output?

- *Cool peripheries*: from a low cardiac output state or sympathetic vasoconstriction, compensation for bleeding or poor fluid resuscitation
- *Pulse*: checking for arrhythmias and tachycardia suggesting bleeding
- *Blood pressure*: may be too low to provide an adequate renal perfusion pressure (NB. a normal BP may be too low to provide adequate renal perfusion in the chronically hypertensive patient)

- *Central venous pressure (CVP)*: if present, provides a useful measurement of filling
- *Dry mouth*: suggests dehydration
- *Distended bladder*: as the urinary catheter may be blocked
- *Drains*: for bleeding losses
- *Drug chart*: for presence of nephrotoxic agents, e.g. aminoglycosides, non-steroidal anti-inflammatory drugs (NSAIDs)
- *Fluid balance chart*: complete anuria suggests catheter obstruction

What is the main risk of ignoring poor urine output?

Persisting renal ischaemia may lead to acute tubular necrosis and established acute kidney injury (AKI). For this reason, post-operative oliguria must be managed in good time.

What investigations would you perform and why?

Investigations serve two main purposes

- To establish the cause for the oliguria
- To determine the effect on the kidney, e.g. is this problem reversible or is there established renal failure?

Some investigations

- *Serum urea and electrolytes (U&Es)*: elevated creatinine shows decreased renal function, and elevated urea is a marker for dehydration
- *Urine sodium and osmolality*: both are indicators of adequate tubular function

- *Other tests*: ECG if a myocardial infarction is suspected, and renal US if obstruction is suspected

How could you tell that the patient has developed acute renal failure?

In the case of oliguria due to acute tubular necrosis, the renal tubules lose their ability to

- Concentrate the urine
- Retain sodium

Thus, certain investigations can be devised to determine if there is tubular dysfunction

Table 5.1

	Acute tubular necrosis (ATN)	Pre-renal failure
Urine Na	>20	<40
Urine osmolality	<500	>350
Urine: plasma osmolality ratio	<1.2	>1.2

How would you manage patients with poor urine output?

Management of these patients must be rapid to prevent AKI

- Give the urinary catheter a flush to resolve any obstruction
- Stop nephrotoxic drugs until the state of oliguria has been resolved
- Give a bolus of colloid or crystalloid, e.g. 250–500 ml of gelofusin, to determine if adequate filling is required. The

response of the CVP to this bolus is also a useful indicator of the circulating volume

- Ensure a good cardiac output, e.g. if the patient is being epicardially paced, the rate may be increased
- If the patient is well filled, small boluses of 10 mg furosemide IV may be given, progressing to an infusion
- Diuretics and inotropes, e.g. dopamine, although increasing the urine output, have not been shown to reduce the risk of progression to acute kidney injury
- Dopamine acts locally to increase the renal blood flow but also has a direct inotropic effect, increasing the cardiac output and renal perfusion pressure
- Renal support in the form of dialysis or haemofiltration may also be required

Renal failure: acute kidney injury (AKI)

What is the definition of acute kidney injury?

The term acute kidney injury has replaced acute renal failure and is an abrupt reduction of kidney function to excrete nitrogenous and other waste products of metabolism in <48 hours. It is, therefore, a biochemical diagnosis loosely defined as an absolute increase in serum creatinine of more than $\geq 26.4 \ \mu mol/L$, a 1.5 factor increase in serum creatinine from baseline or a documented oliguria of <30 ml/kg/h for >6 hours.

How are the causes classified?

The causes may be pre-renal, renal and post-renal, and 5–20% of critically ill patients develop AKI.

What are the major renal causes of acute kidney injury?

- Acute tubular necrosis
- Glomerulonephritis
- Tubulointerstitial nephritis
- Bilateral cortical necrosis
- Renovascular
  - Vasculitis
  - Renal artery thrombosis
- Hepatorenal syndrome, e.g. in liver failure

What is acute tubular necrosis?

Acute tubular necrosis is renal failure resulting from injury to the tubular epithelial cells, and is the most important cause of acute kidney injury. There are two types

- *Ischaemic injury*: following any cause of shock, which results in a fall in renal perfusion pressure and oxygenation
- *Nephrogenic injury*: from drugs (aminoglycosides, paracetamol), toxins (heavy metals, organic solvents), or myoglobin (from rhabdomyolysis)

What are the major post-renal causes?

- Acute obstruction from urinary calculi
- Obstruction from tumours arising from the renal parenchyma or transitional epithelium of the pelvicalyceal system
- Extrinsic compression from pelvic tumours
- Iatrogenic injury, e.g. inadvertent damage to the ureters during colorectal surgery

- Prostatic enlargement and obstruction
- Increased intra-abdominal pressure ($>30\,cmH_2O$)

Which part of the kidney is the most poorly perfused?

The renal medulla is poorly perfused compared to the cortex. This ensures the medullary interstitial concentration gradient formed by the tubular counter current multiplier is preserved and maintained.

Which part of the nephron is the most susceptible to ischaemic injury and why?

The cells of the thick ascending limb are the most susceptible to ischaemic injury for two important reasons

- The cells reside in the medulla, which has poorer oxygenation than the cortex
- The active Na^+ and K^+ ATPase pumps on the cell membrane have a high oxygen demand

What are the basic steps in the pathogenesis of acute kidney injury?

The basic steps in the pathogenesis are

- *Vasoconstriction*: this is a compensatory response to a fall in the renal perfusion pressure, of the efferent arteriole. This maintains capillary filtration pressure, at the expense of reducing blood supply to the tubules perfused by the efferent arteriole. Worsening cortical and medullary ischaemia results

- *Obstruction*: tubular cell ischaemia and necrosis leads to cells being shed into the tubular lumen, causing obstruction
- *Pressure changes*: obstruction causes a back leak of tubular fluid into the parenchyma, increasing the interstitial hydrostatic pressure

These act in concert to reduce tubular fluid reabsorption, worsening the oliguria.

Name some common drugs of surgical importance that may exacerbate or cause acute kidney injury

- *Paracetamol*: overdose is a known cause of acute tubular necrosis
- *Non-steroidal anti-inflammatory drugs (NSAIDs)*: can lead to renal failure by reducing the renal protective effects of prostaglandins during renal ischaemia
- *Aminoglycosides*: a potent cause of acute tubular necrosis, e.g. gentamicin
- *Penicillins*: can cause tubulointerstitial nephritis
- *Furosemide*: can lead to tubulointerstitial nephritis
- *Dextran 40*: a colloid sometimes used during fluid resuscitation

How is acute kidney injury recognised?

Acute kidney injury is a biochemical diagnosis

- Oliguria (<400 ml/day) may or may not be present
- Biochemical markers of reduced glomerular filtration rate (GFR), e.g. acutely elevated serum urea and creatinine, compared to baseline

- Biochemical markers of diminished electrolyte homeostasis, e.g. hyponatraemia, hyperkalaemia, metabolic acidosis, hypocalcaemia
- Changes in the composition of the urine compared to the plasma (*see* Oliguria: Low Urine Output state)

How may it be distinguished from chronic kidney disease?

It may sometimes be difficult to distinguish from pre-existing chronic kidney disease, but some clues may be gathered from different sources

- *Clinical*: signs and symptoms of chronic kidney disease, e.g. skin pigmentation, chronic anaemia, pruritis or nocturia, may be present
- *Biochemical*: previous blood results may suggest long-term renal suppression or deterioration
- *Radiological*: in chronic kidney disease, ultrasound examination reveals small or scarred kidneys

What are the two most important life-threatening complications?

- *Acute pulmonary oedema*: due to fluid retention from over-hydration
- *Hyperkalaemia*: leading to metabolic acidosis and cardiac arrhythmias

Both may require urgent dialysis as part of the management.

What are the principles of management of established acute kidney injury?

- *Drugs*: stop all nephrotoxic agents and careful use of other drugs that undergo renal excretion

- *Fluid resuscitation*: this must be judicious to ensure that the patient is not tipped into acute pulmonary oedema. Adequate fluid balance requires a daily fluid balance chart, and daily examination and weighing of the patient
- *Nutritional support*: best performed by the enteral route, paying special attention to the protein input
- *Managing underlying disease*: e.g. obstruction, sepsis, glomerulonephritis
- *Renal replacement therapies (RRTs)*: e.g. haemodialysis, peritoneal dialysis, haemofiltration

Complications need to be managed, e.g. prophylaxis for GI bleeding with the use of H^+ antagonists, which can increase the urea load.

What is the prognosis of acute kidney injury?

The mortality of isolated renal failure is ~5–10%. However, depending on the cause, there is often a good recovery of renal function within several weeks.

Renal failure: chronic kidney disease (CKD)

What is the definition of chronic kidney disease (CKD)?

CKD is kidney damage for >3 months based on proven structural and functional abnormalities. It rarely occurs in isolation, being mostly caused by hypertension and diabetes in the Western world, progressing to end-stage renal failure (ESRF) in 4% over a 5-year period.

What is the normal level of serum creatinine?

60–120 μmol/L (micromoles). NB. Units are given as μmols and not mmols.

What then is creatinine?

Creatinine is creatine minus a water molecule (i.e. anhydride of creatine). It is formed in muscle by the non-enzymatic and irreversible degradation of creatine phosphate.

Why is the serum creatinine a better indicator of renal function than serum urea concentration?

Serum urea is a poor indicator of the GFR as ~50% of filtered urea undergoes reabsorption at the tubules. This underestimates the GFR. Also, the daily production of urea is more variable than creatinine.

What is the prevalence of chronic kidney disease and how is it classified?

The prevalence is ~4.1% in those aged 18 years and over in England (not age adjusted). Classification is based on the presence of kidney damage and GFR (ml/min/1.73m^2) irrespective of the diagnosis

- *Stage 1 (GFR >90)*: normal or increased GFR
- *Stage 2 (GFR 60–89)*: slight decrease in GFR and other evidence of damage to the kidneys
- *Stage 3A (GFR 45–59)*: moderate decrease in GFR, with or without evidence of other kidney damage
- *Stage 3B (GFR 30–44)*: moderate decrease in GFR, with or without evidence of other kidney damage
- *Stage 4 (GFR 15–29)*: severe decrease in GFR, with or without evidence of other kidney damage
- *Stage 5 (GFR <15)*: established renal failure

Give some causes for chronic kidney disease

The causes may be classified under a number of different headings

- *Congenital*: e.g. polycystic kidney disease
- *Glomerular disease*: including chronic glomerulonephritis, diabetes mellitus, amyloidosis
- *Renovascular*: from hypertensive nephrosclerosis, chronic vasculitis, e.g. SLE
- *Tubular/interstitial*: due to chronic tubulointerstitial nephritis, chronic pyelonephritis
- *Chronic outflow obstruction*: e.g. urinary tract calculi, prostatic enlargement, pelvic tumours

What are the clinical features and the complications of chronic kidney disease?

Clinical signs and symptoms may not be seen until the GFR is <15% of normal (Stage 5)

- *Hypertension*: from fluid retention
- *Polyuria and nocturia*: due to osmotic diuresis caused by uraemia
- *Oedema*: due to a combination of fluid retention and proteinuria
- *Features of uraemia*: circulating uraemic toxins, e.g. organic acids, lead to skin pigmentation, anorexia, nausea, malaise and constipation
- *Haematological*: a normocytic, normochromic anaemia develops leading to lethargy and dypsnoea

- *Renal osteodystrophy*: due to a combination of osteomalacia, osteitis fibrosa cystica and osteosclerosis. This can lead to secondary hyperparathyroidism, metastatic calcifications, bone pain and pathological fractures
- *Neurological*: myoclonic twitches, muscle cramps, mental slowing

Some complications are

- *Cardiac*: uraemic cardiomyopathy
- *Pericardial*: uraemic pericarditis
- *Respiratory*: pulmonary oedema
- *Vascular*: peripheral vascular disease due to a combination of hyperlipidaemia and hypertension
- *Haematological*: bleeding tendency due to platelet dysfunction

Run through the list of acid–base and electrolyte disturbances that are seen
- Hyponatraemia
- Hyperkalaemia
- Hypocalcaemia
- Hyperphosphataemia

This produces a resultant metabolic acidosis (and an increased anion gap), resulting in a reduced serum bicarbonate and an increased serum creatinine, indicating a chronic decline in function.

What is the pathophysiology of renal osteodystrophy?
There are a number of pathological processes that lead to bone disease

- Reduced renal production of 1-α-hydroxylase results in a reduction of calcitriol (1,25 dihydroxy-vitamin D_3)
- This leads to secondary hyperparathyroidism
- Hyperparathyroidism increases bone resorption, bone cyst formation and osteitis fibrosa cystica
- Hyperphosphataemia develops as a direct consequence of reduced renal function
- Deficiency of 1,25 dihydroxy-vitamin D_3 reduces bone mineralisation with resulting osteomalacia

Why are uraemic patients anaemic?

Uraemic patients may develop a normocytic, normochromic anaemia for a number of reasons

- Deficiency of erythropoietin (most important cause)
- Presence of circulating bone marrow toxins
- Bone marrow fibrosis during osteitis fibrosa cystica
- Increased red cell fragility caused by uraemic toxins

What would you expect to find when you examine a patient with chronic kidney disease?

- The patient may be tachypnoeic from metabolic acidosis, e.g. Kussmaul's
- Pigmentation of the skin as a direct effect of uraemia. There may also be scratch marks on the skin from uraemic pruritis
- Hands may have brown discolouration in the fingernails, or exhibit a fistula at the wrist for dialysis
- The abdomen may reveal the scar from a previous renal transplant

- Hypertension may develop due to fluid overload, and there may be a pericardial friction rub from uraemic pericarditis. Peripherally, pitting oedema is common
- Peripheral neuropathy also develops
- Features of the underlying causes, palpable kidneys in polycystic disease, peripheral vascular disease in diabetes mellitus

How is chronic kidney disease managed?

The principles of management are

- There is optimisation of bone mineralisation and improvement of hypocalcaemia, so patients are given α-calcidol and calcitriol
- The hyperphosphataemia can be managed using gut phosphate binders, e.g. Calcichew®
- Anaemia can be reversed with the use of subcutaneous recombinant human erythropoietin
- Hypertension is generally managed using the same agents as those with normal renal function. High-dose loop diuretics are in common use, e.g. furosemide to keep BP <140/85 mmHg
- Dietary considerations include restricting the protein intake to reduce urea production. Sodium restriction helps to limit fluid overload. Potassium restriction is also required. Vitamin supplements replace the water-soluble vitamins lost during dialysis
- Fluid restriction limits the development of oedema

- Other aspects of management includes control of nausea, laxatives for constipation
- ESRF requires haemodialysis for renal transplantation

Other systemic processes

Burns

How common are burn injuries in the UK?

In the UK, burns account for 0.29 per 1000 of hospital admissions and 300 deaths per annum, and tend to occur in the old, the young and the unlucky.

What types of burns are there?

Burns may be

- Thermal, due to extreme heat and cold
- Electrical
- Chemical, due to caustic substances, e.g. acids

What criteria may be used for the assessment of thermal burns?

Burns are assessed by their extent on the body and their depth of skin penetration

- *Extent*: this is described in terms of the percentage (%) body surface area (BSA) covered according to the Wallace rule of 9s, e.g. the palm is equivalent to 1%, anterior and posterior trunk 18%, head and arms 9%, legs 18% and genitalia 1%

- *Depth*: may be superficial, superficial dermal, mid-dermal, deep dermal and full thickness. The clinical determinants of the depth are
  - Colour: e.g. red, pale pink, dark pink, fixed staining, yellow. The erythema is prominent in superficial burns
  - Capillary refill time (CRT): normal, reduced, absent
  - Sensation: burns are painful in areas, where there is no deep dermal, full thickness penetration
  - Blisters: present in superficial dermal and mid-dermal burns
  - Healing: occurs in superficial but not deep and full thickness burns
  - Texture: leathery skin seen with full thickness burns

Why are burns patients susceptible to respiratory complications?

- There may be a thermal injury to the nose or oropharynx with upper airway oedema
- Smoke inhalation can lead to hypoxia with pulmonary oedema from ARDS
- Inhalation of carbon monoxide
- Inhalation of other toxic gases such as cyanide, or the oxides of sulphur and nitrogen
- Circumferential burns of the chest may restrict respiration
- Aggressive fluid resuscitation may produce pulmonary oedema
- A superadded chest infection may complicate pulmonary oedema

Why is carbon monoxide (CO) toxic?

- Its affinity for haemoglobin (forming carboxyhaemoglobin) is ~250 times greater than that of oxygen, and it has a long half-life of 250 minutes (breathing room air) and 40 minutes (breathing 100% oxygen)
- Consequently, the oxygen dissociation curve is shifted to the left with poor oxygenation of the tissues
- It also binds to some of the respiratory chain enzymes, such as cytochrome oxidase, therefore affecting oxygen utilisation at the cellular level
- CO levels of 0–15% may be present in smokers, 15–20% produces headache and confusion, 20–40% results in hallucinations and ataxia, and levels >60% are fatal

CO poisoning should be treated with 100% humidified oxygen, and this should be continued for 48 hours as a secondary release of CO occurs from the cytochrome system.

When would you become suspicious of an impending respiratory problem?

- Fire in a confined space
- Soot at the mouth or in the sputum
- Burns on the face, singeing of the eyebrows and nasal hair
- Hoarse voice, stridor and a brassy cough
- Swollen upper airways
- Serum carboxyhaemoglobin >10%

Why are burns patients susceptible to acute kidney injury?

- Hypovolaemia from plasma loss reduces the renal perfusion pressure, precipitating the development of acute tubular necrosis

- Circulating myoglobin produces rhabdomyolysis, resulting in tubular injury and acute tubular necrosis
- Acute kidney injury may occur as a consequence of sepsis and the systemic inflammatory response syndrome (SIRS)

What are the other systemic complications of severe burns?

Aside from respiratory and renal failure, the other systematic complications are

- '*Burns shock*', which is hypovolaemic shock due to plasma loss following loss of skin cover. This leads to hypotension, tachycardia, increased systemic vascular resistance and a fall in cardiac output
- Electrolyte disturbances, including hypo- or hypernatraemia, hyperkalaemia, hypocalcaemia
- Hypothermia following loss of skin cover; convection heaters may be used
- Systemic inflammatory response syndrome (SIRS) that can lead to multi-organ dysfunction and high mortality
- Generalised sepsis from organisms that include Clostridia. The features indicating sepsis may be indistinguishable from other causes of SIRS
- Gastric ulceration as part of the stress response
- Coagulopathy due to disseminated intravascular coagulation and hypothermia
- Haemolysis leading to haemoglobinuria and anaemia

Describe the principles behind the early management

Management of burns involves immediate ABCDE assessment and adherence to the ATLS® system of trauma care involving identification of any other injuries

- *Airway*: signs of an impending respiratory problem require intubation (*see* above)
- *Breathing*: looking for the presence of respiratory distress, which may not be initially evident. High-flow oxygen is given. Early intubation and ventilation may again be required
- *Circulation*: monitoring of fluid therapy and cardiovascular function necessitates the insertion of a central venous catheter (CVC). The arterial pressure is supported with IV fluids
- *Renal*: this involves maintenance of the renal perfusion pressure with IV fluids. Given the added risk of rhabdomyolysis, a urinary catheter should be inserted and the urine output maintained >0.5 ml/kg/h
- *Thermoregulation*: preventing hypothermia using convection heaters and a warm ambient temperature. This also helps to control the hypermetabolic state
- *Gastrointestinal*: stress ulcer prophylaxis is commenced, e.g. sucralfate
- *Surgery*: this has a role in the emergency management of constricting circumferential thoracic eschars that can cause respiratory embarrassment, or a tracheostomy to manage airway difficulties

It is also important to provide adequate analgesia, e.g. IV opioids may be required, and antibiotics if a proven source of sepsis is identified or the mechanism of injury has a high index of clinical suspicion of potential infection.

How much fluid would you give?

There are a number of formulae to determine the rate and level of fluid replacement. Ultimately, the amount of fluid given depends on the clinical situation

- IV fluids are commenced if >15% adult or >10% paediatric BSA. Deeper and more extensive burns may require a blood transfusion, especially in the context of other injuries
- The Parkland formula (adopted by the ATLS® protocol) is 2–4 ml/kg/% burn in the first 24 hours, half of this is to be given in the first 8 hours and the second half is given in the next 16 hours
- The Muir-Barclay formula divides fluid administration into a number of discrete time periods. The amount of fluid given in each period is 0.5 ml/kg/% burn of colloid per unit time. The first 24 hours is divided into periods of 4, 4, 4, 6, 6 and 12 hours

The fluids should be estimated from the time of the burn, and do not include maintenance fluids, and the urine output should be kept at >0.5 ml/kg/h. Inhalational and crush injuries require greater amounts of fluid.

How do you assess the adequacy of fluid therapy?

A number of clinical parameters may be used

- Clinical measures of the cardiac index includes peripheral warmth, capillary refill time and urine output
- Central venous pressure and its response to fluid challenges
- Core temperature, e.g. rectal temperature
- Haematocrit (Hct), which determines the plasma volume and the red cell mass. This is unreliable if there has been a recent transfusion or haemolysis

What are the nutritional requirements?

The calorific requirements should be commenced at an early stage and preferably enteral

- *Curreri formula*: for adults it is 25 kcal/kg + 40 kcal/%BSA, and for children it is 40–60 kcal/kg/%BSA. The calorie:nitrogen ratio should be 150:1

Nutrition: basic concepts

Describe how the state of nutrition may be assessed

There are many methods of assessing the nutritional state but none of them completely satisfactory

- Anthropometric measures
  - Height, weight and body mass index (BMI), e.g. weight (kg)/height(m^2)
  - Fat measure indices, e.g. triceps skin-fold thickness
  - Lean muscle indices, e.g. mid-arm circumference
- Biochemical indices
  - *Serum proteins*: e.g. albumin, more of a late marker because of the long half-life ($t_{\frac{1}{2}}$ 20 days). Other states of

critical illness may also affect the level. Other proteins that have been measured include pre-albumin, transferrin and retinol, all of which may be affected by the stress response

- *24-hour urinary creatinine*: as a measure of the protein turnover
- Immunological indices
  - Total lymphocyte count
  - Immune function, e.g. tuberculin skin test, response to mitogens. However, these are non-specific
- Clinical markers
  - Physical appearance
  - Hand-grip strength
  - Pulmonary function tests, e.g. vital capacity

From which sources may the energy requirements be satisfied? How much energy does each of these provide?

The predominant sources of energy are from carbohydrates and lipid, but protein catabolism also yields energy

- Fats provide 9.3 kcal/g of energy
- Glucose provides 4.1 kcal/g of energy
- Protein provides 4.1 kcal/g of energy

Define the respiratory quotient

This is defined as 'the ratio of the volume of the CO_2 produced to the volume of oxygen consumed for the oxidation of a given amount of nutrient'. Respiratory quotients for the oxidation of nutrients are

- Carbohydrate: 1.0

- Fat: 0.70
- Protein: 0.80

What are the disadvantages of using glucose as the main energy source? How can this be overcome?

The problems of glucose are

- *Glucose intolerance*: as part of the stress response, critically unwell patients are often in a state of hyperglycaemia and glucose intolerance. Therefore, if glucose is the only source of energy, patients will not receive their required daily amount due to poor utilisation of their energy source
- *Fatty liver*: the excess glucose occurring as a consequence of the above is converted to lipid in the liver, leading to fatty change. This may derange the liver function tests
- *Respiratory failure*: the extra CO_2 released upon oxidation of the glucose may lead to respiratory failure and increased ventilatory requirements

Relying solely on glucose may lead to a deficiency of the essential fatty acids. Therefore, ~50% of the total energy requirement must be provided by fat. Conversely, too little glucose leads to hypoglycaemia and the stimulation of ketogenesis.

What is the recommended daily intake of protein and nitrogen?

The recommended daily intake of protein is 0.8 g/kg/day and that of nitrogen is 0.15 g/kg/day. Note that these values increase in the catabolic state of critical illness.

How much protein provides 1 g of nitrogen?

6.25 g of protein yields 1 g of nitrogen.

What is an essential amino acid? Give examples

The essential amino acids are those that cannot be synthesised in the body and have to be ingested in the diet. They include: histidine, isoleucine, leucine, lysine, methionine, phenylalanine, threonine, tryptophan and valine.

Give some examples of essential minerals (elements)

The essential elements include calcium, chlorine, chromium, copper, iodine, iron, magnesium, manganese, molybdenum, phosphorus, potassium, selenium, sodium and zinc.

What are the fat-soluble vitamins, and what are they used for?

- *Vitamin A*: important for cell membrane stabilisation and retinal function
- *Vitamin D*: for calcium homeostasis and bone mineralisation
- *Vitamin E*: acts as a free radical scavenger
- *Vitamin K*: involved in the γ-carboxylation of glutamic acid residues of Factors II, VII, IX and X during blood coagulation

What are the names of the vitamin B group? Which diseases occur when there is a deficiency?

The B group of vitamins, which are all water soluble, are composed of

- *Vitamin B$_1$ (thiamine)*: deficiency leads to beriberi or Wernicke's encephalopathy

- *Vitamin B_2 (riboflavin)*: deficiency leads to a syndrome of glossitis, angular stomatitis and cheilosis
- *Vitamin B_3 (niacin)*: deficiency leads to pellagra
- *Vitamin B_5 (panthothenic acid)*: deficiency can lead to acne and parathesia
- *Vitamin B_6 (pyridoxine)*: deficiency leads to stomatitis and peripheral neuropathy
- *Vitamin B_7 (biotin)*: deficiency rarely occurs in isolation, but can lead to reduced immune function
- *Vitamin B_9 (folate)*: deficiency leads to macrocytic anaemia and neural tube defects in pregnancy
- *Vitamin B_{12} (cobalamin)*: deficiency produces megaloblastic anaemia, peripheral neuropathy

What are the functions of vitamin C?

Vitamin C is another of the water-soluble vitamins and is important for

- Hydroxylation of proline and lysine residues during collagen synthesis
- Iron absorption in the gut
- Synthesis of adrenaline from tyrosine
- Antioxidant functions

Nutrition: enteral

What are the indications for enteral nutrition?

Enteral feeding should be provided for those patients with a functionally intact GI system that cannot meet their daily nutritional requirements. If the gut works, use it.

By which routes may enteral nutrition be administered?

- *Oral nutritional supplementation*: taken between meals, being mainly milk or soya protein based
- *Nasoenteric feeding*: either into the stomach (nasogastric, NG) or jejunum (nasojejunal, NJ) using a fine-bore feeding tube to minimise oesophageal irritation. NJ feeding bypasses the stomach for those with impaired gastric motility and reduces pancreatic stimulation in those with acute pancreatitis. Therefore, it has reduced the risk of pulmonary aspiration
- *Gastrostomy*: this may be placed during surgery or percutaneously by endoscopic or fluoroscopic techniques, e.g. percutaneous endoscopic gastrostomy (PEG), radiologically inserted gastrostomy (RIG). It is suitable for prolonged feeding, particularly in those with head injuries or other neurological deficits affecting coordinated swallowing
- *Jejunostomy*: this is usually placed at laparotomy in those in whom prolonged feeding is anticipated. The tube is sutured to the anti-mesenteric side of the jejunum. Note that this bypasses the pancreas and biliary tree and reduces the risk of aspiration

What is the difference between a polymeric and elemental diet?

A polymeric diet is given to those with well-functioning GI tracts, unlike elemental diets, which are reserved for those with malabsorption, e.g. short bowel syndrome. With polymeric diets, whole protein is used as the source of nitrogen, but for elemental diets, free amino acids or oligopeptides are used.

Glucose polymers and long chain triglycerides are the source of carbohydrate and fat, respectively, for elemental diets.

What other enteral diets are available?
- *Modular diets*: this diet has been enriched in a particular nutrient for the requirement of specific patients
- *Special formulation diets*: these are arranged for specific diseases, e.g. ventilated patients are given a diet rich in fat as the main energy source as opposed to glucose, in order to reduce CO_2 generation during metabolism

Why should gastrically fed patients be given a break from feeding at some point during a 24 hour period?
There are two main reasons why gastric feeding is not continuous

- *Aspiration*: feeding without a break encourages bacterial colonisation of the stomach. This increases the risk of developing nosocomial pneumonia if there is aspiration
- *Diarrhoea*: continuous intragastric feeding causes a secretory response from the ascending colon leading to diarrhoea. This may be due to the loss of the normal cephalic phase of secretion

What happens to the bowel in those who are not fed enterally?
It is known that absence of enteral feeding leads to atrophic changes in the intestinal mucosa. This is because local

hormonal release in response to food stimulates the release of enzymes necessary for mucosal integrity.

What is the result of mucosal atrophy?

- Loss of cellular adhesion and development of cellular channels
- Translocation of bacteria across the bowel wall into the systemic circulation is encouraged. This can lead to sepsis, or perpetuation of the systemic inflammatory response syndrome (SIRS) in the critically ill

Give some complications associated with enteral feeding

- Tube displacement, e.g. jejunal migration can lead to diarrhoea
- Infection around a gastrostomy or jejunostomy wound
- Re-feeding syndrome leads to hypophosphataemia in the malnourished, thrombocytopaenia and confusion
- Hyperkalaemia in those with renal impairment
- Hyperglycaemia in those with the reduced glucose tolerance of the critically ill

Nutrition: total parenteral (TPN)

What are the indications for TPN?

- General critical illness
  - Severe malnourishment with >10% loss of weight
  - Multiple trauma
  - Sepsis/multi-system failure
  - Severe burns

- Gut problems
    - Enterocutaneous fistula
    - Short bowel syndrome
    - Inflammatory bowel disease
    - Radiation enteritis

Which is the absolute indication for TPN?

The most important indication is the presence of an enterocutaneous fistula.

How is TPN administered?

The high osmolality of the mixture causes irritation to small vessels, so that it is generally given through a central vein, e.g. tunnelled subclavian line. If it is to be given through a peripheral vein, e.g. through a peripherally inserted central catheter (PICC), it must be given as a solution of osmolality of <900 mOsm/L.

What are the basic components of a TPN regimen?

The basic components are water, carbohydrate, protein, lipid, vitamins and trace elements. Various drugs may also be added, such as ranitidine and insulin.

How is TPN monitored?

Monitoring involves nutritional status and biochemical markers, and depending on the clinical context and risk of re-feeding syndrome and other complications, includes glucose, serum electrolytes, urea and creatinine, albumin and total protein, calcium, magnesium, phosphate and liver function tests. These measurements can be twice daily, daily, twice weekly or weekly.

Why does liver function need to be monitored?

TPN can cause a derangement of the liver function tests secondary to enzyme induction caused by amino acid imbalances. Also, it can cause fatty change, non-alcoholic fatty liver disease, intrahepatic cholestasis, cholecystitis and cholelithiasis.

What are the metabolic complications?

- Hypo- and hyperglycaemia
- Hyperlipidaemia
- Hyperchloraemic metabolic acidosis (if there is an excess of chloride)
- Hyperammoniaemia, e.g. if there is liver disease, or a deficiency of L-glutamine and arginine
- Essential fatty acid deficiency
- Ventilatory problems due to excess production of CO_2 if too much glucose is used in the mixture. In the ventilated critically ill patient, the amount of glucose given in 24 hours may have to be restricted to 5 g/kg

Other complications include infection, from line sepsis, and thromboembolic phenomena, due to micro-embolic formation at the IV cannula site. The most potent risk is that of the re-feeding syndrome, particularly in the chronically malnourished.

Rhabdomyolysis

What is myoglobin composed of and what is its function?
Myoglobin, a respiratory pigment found in cardiac and skeletal muscle, is composed of a single globin chain of 8 α-helical regions with a single haem component. It is a ready source of oxygen for muscle during times of increased activity.

How does the O_2 dissociation curve for myoglobin differ from that of haemoglobin, and what accounts for this difference?
The shape of the dissociation curve for myoglobin is hyperbolic, as opposed to sigmoidal for haemoglobin. Unlike haemoglobin, CO_2 or pH does not affect the curve and myoglobin, consisting of only one globin chain and haem molecule, does not exhibit these interactions caused by multiple globin chains and haem molecules.

What is rhabdomyolysis?
Rhabdomyolysis is a clinical syndrome caused by the release of potentially toxic muscle cell components into the circulation. It has many triggers, including trauma, drugs, metabolic and congenital conditions.

What kinds of traumatic insult can trigger this off?
Trauma to muscle cell integrity may be caused by

- Blunt trauma to skeletal muscle, e.g. crush injury
- Prolonged immobilisation on a hard surface

- Massive burns
- Strenuous and prolonged spontaneous exercise, e.g. marathon running
- Hypothermia
- Hyperthermia due to malignant hyperpyrexia
- Acute ischaemic and reperfusion injury, e.g. clamp on an artery during surgery
- Drugs, e.g. statins, fibrates, alcohol, neuroleptic malignant syndrome

What complications may it lead to?

In the severest form, it may be complicated by

- *Acute kidney injury (AKI)*: may develop in up to 30% of those with rhabdomyolysis
- *Disseminated intravascular coagulation (DIC)*: due to pathological activation of the coagulation cascade by the released muscle compounds
- *Metabolic disturbances*: due to electrolyte disturbances, e.g. hyperkalaemia from haemolysis and AKI
- *Compartment syndrome*: muscle injury may be associated with a rise in the intracompartmental pressure leading to worsening ischaemia and renal perfusion pressure (AKI)
- *Hypovolaemia*: due to haemorrhage into the necrotic muscle. This may exacerbate the diminished renal function

List the associated electrolyte disturbances

Disturbances include

- Hyperkalaemia (and metabolic acidosis with an increased anion gap)
- Hypocalcaemia
- Hyperphosphataemia
- Hyperuricaemia

What is the basic mechanism for the development of acute kidney injury in rhabdomyolysis?
The exact mechanism is not fully understood but may involve ischaemic tubular injury caused by myoglobin and its breakdown products accumulating in the renal tubules.

How is the diagnosis of rhabdomyolysis confirmed?
There is an elevated plasma creatinine kinase (CK) >1000 U/L (often >10 000 U/L). This is over five times the upper limit of normal. It has several isoenzymes, e.g. CK-MB, and a myocardial infarction needs to be excluded, but CK-MM is specific to skeletal muscle injury. Other tests include

- Elevated serum lactate dehydrogenase (LDH)
- Elevated serum creatinine
- Myoglobinuria suggested by positive dipstick to blood in the absence of haemoglobinuria (red cells on microscopy)

The presence of dark urine due to the presence of myoglobin occurs when urinary myoglobin exceeds 250 μg/ml, which corresponds to ~100 g of muscle destruction. All of these have to be taken in the context of a potential triggering factor.

What are the principles of management of a patient who has developed rhabdomyolysis following trauma?

The principle of therapy is largely supportive, managing complications and ensuring adequate renal function. In the context of trauma, this should be according to the ATLS® protocol

- *Fluid resuscitation*: ensure good hydration to support urine output >300 ml/h using IV crystalloid until myoglobinuria has ceased. Diuretics, e.g. mannitol, may also be used for this end
- *Alkalinisation*: sodium bicarbonate infusion has been used to limit myoglobin-induced tubular injury in the presence of acidic urine. It alkalinises the urine >6.5 pH
- *Electrolyte disturbances*: particularly hyperkalaemia caused by the release of potassium by the injured muscle and exacerbated by metabolic acidosis. It should be managed promptly (*see* Electrolyte Balance: Potassium). If renal function worsens, dialysis or haemofiltration may have to be performed

In most cases, a full renal recovery is likely.

What are the clinical features of compartment syndrome?

For compartment syndrome of the limbs

- *Worsening pain*: this may be out of proportion to the injury
- *Paraesthesia*: especially loss of two-point tactile discrimination

Clinical signs are

- Tense and swollen compartments
- Sensory loss
- Pain on passive stretching
- Loss of regional pulses, which is a late sign

What levels of compartmental pressure may lead to compartment syndrome?

The first symptoms of pain and paraesthesia appear at compartmental pressures of 20–30 mmHg. Normal resting pressure is 0–8 mmHg.

What is the surgical management of compartment syndrome?

The primary treatment is decompression fasciotomy before the onset of necrosis and subsequent contracture. Some advocate a pressure of >30 mmHg as being the cut-off for fasciotomy, while others rely on the relationship of the compartmental pressure to the diastolic pressure.

Systemic response to trauma

Give some examples of stimuli that may activate the systemic stress response

- Trauma resulting in pain and tissue injury
- Surgery
- Infection, e.g. endotoxin is a powerful stimulus
- Hypothermia
- Severe acid–base disturbances
- Acute hypoglycaemia

Which four physiological systems are involved in coordinating the systemic stress response?

- *Sympathetic nervous system*: producing changes in the cardiovascular, endocrine and metabolic systems, e.g. promotes hyperglycaemia and activation of the renin–angiotensin–aldosterone (RAA) system
- *Endocrine system*: glucocorticoid release is stimulated by ACTH following the stress stimulus. Their plasma levels remain elevated for as long as the stimulus is present. Other hormones that are increased during the response are glucagon, thyroxine, growth hormone, histamine and endogenous opioids
- *Acute phase response*: with the release of cytokines, prostaglandins, leucotrienes and kinins
- *Microcirculatory system*: with changes in the vascular tone and permeability affecting tissue oxygen delivery. Vasoactive mediators such as nitric oxide, prostaglandins and platelet-activating factor induce vasodilatation and increased capillary permeability

What are the main glucocorticoids in the body? Give some examples of some of their systemic effects

The two main active glucocorticoids in the body are cortisol and corticosterone. Their effects are

- Metabolic
  - *Glucose metabolism*: stimulation of gluconeogenesis and peripheral antagonism of insulin leads to hyperglycaemia and glucose intolerance

- *Protein*: increased uptake of amino acids into the liver and promotion of protein catabolism in the peripheral tissues, such as muscle
  - *Lipid*: stimulation of lipolysis in adipose tissue
- Endocrine
  - *Mineralocorticoid activity*: promoting sodium and water retention with loss of potassium, all being mediated at the renal level

Coordination of the stress response enables anti-inflammatory, immunosuppressive and anti-allergic actions to also occur. This also has a permissive effect on the actions of other hormones.

Draw a diagram showing the change in the basal metabolic rate following a traumatic insult to the body

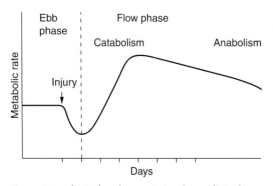

Figure 5.1 Adapted with permission from *Clinical Surgery in General*, 3rd edn. Edited by Kirk, Mansfield and Cochrane (1999), p. 305. Published by Churchill Livingstone, ISBN 0443062196.

What happens during the two phases of the metabolic response?

- *Ebb phase*: there is a reduction in the metabolic rate in the 24 hours following the stimulus
- *Flow phase*: an increase in the metabolic rate, with generalised catabolism, negative nitrogen balance and glucose intolerance. The degree of metabolic increase depends on the type of initiating insult

Why is there a fall in the urine output immediately following a traumatic insult such as surgery? When does this resolve?

Following surgery, there is activation of the RAA system and increased release of antidiuretic hormone as part of the response. Thus, the urine output may remain low despite adequate volume replacement. It resolves usually in 24 hours, but sodium retention may persist for several days.

Why may metabolic alkalosis develop and what effect does this have on oxygen delivery to the tissues?

The mineralocorticoid effects of cortisol and aldosterone promote sodium retention at the expense of potassium. Loss of potassium can lead to a metabolic alkalosis. With the reduction of H^+ that defines metabolic alkalosis, the oxygen dissociation curve is shifted to the left (increased oxygen affinity), reducing tissue oxygen delivery. Note that in the latter stages of the response, if there is a fall in tissue perfusion, then the patient can become acidotic.

What changes may occur in the various organ systems during the systemic stress response?

- *Cardiac*: the cardiac output increases in the initial stages
- *Respiratory*: hyperventilation leads to a respiratory alkalosis. In the latter stages, as part of the systemic inflammatory response syndrome (SIRS), acute lung injury and ARDS may supervene
- *Hepatic*: there is a reduction in the production of albumin
- *Haematological*: there is systemic activation of the coagulation cascade, which if severe enough, can lead to disseminated intravascular coagulation

Bibliography

American College of Surgeons. Thermal injuries. In *Advanced Trauma Life Support*® *(ATLS*®*)*, 9th edn. Chicago, IL, American College of Surgeons; 2012: Chapter 9.

Gupta A, Reilly CS. Fat embolism. Continuing education in anaesthesia. *Critical Care and Pain Journal.* 2007;7(5): 148–51.

NHS Kidney Care. *Kidney Disease: Key Facts and Figures.* 2010: 1–40.

Richards AM, Jackson IT. Burns. In *Key Notes on Plastic Surgery*. Oxford, Blackwell Science; 2002: 273–83.

Intensive care (level 3)

Chapter 6

Intensive care unit (ICU)

Assessment

Agitation and sedation

Give some causes of acute confusion in the post-operative patient

- *Pain (anxiety and disorientation)*: all of these can commonly occur in critically ill patients
- *Sepsis*: systemic infection, or localised to chest, urinary tract, wound, intra-abdominal, intrathoracic, intracranial collection
- *Glycaemic disturbances*: this occurs most commonly with hypoglycaemia, but can occur in hyperglycaemia, e.g. ketoacidosis
- *Metabolic*: electrolyte disturbances can precipitate agitation, most commonly hypo- or hypernatraemia
- *Respiratory*: a compromise in respiratory function can lead to hypoxaemia and hypercarbia. Usual precipitating causes, apart from a chest infection, include acute pulmonary oedema, pneumothorax, pulmonary embolism, sputum retention and subsequent atelectasis

- *Cardiovascular*: low cardiac output state and hypotension from any cause, e.g. bleeding, myocardial infarction, arrhythmia leading to reduced cerebral perfusion
- *Renal*: acute kidney injury and hepatic failure can cause the accumulation of encephalopathic toxins to develop, e.g. uraemia. Urinary retention in the elderly can be a causative factor
- *Fluid imbalance*: both dehydration and water overload can exacerbate the hyponatraemia due to the fluid retention from the stress response to surgery
- *Drugs*: e.g. opiate analgesia, excess sedative drugs, anticholinergics

Which investigations should you perform?

Following a full history and examination investigations include

Bedside investigations

- *Boehringer Mannheim (BM)*: this rapidly assesses if the capillary glucose is low and this provides a value 7% higher than plasma values
- *Arterial blood gas (ABG) analysis*: this determines the base excess and respiratory function, e.g. if hypoxia or hypercarbia is present
- *Electrocardiograph (ECG)*: for arrhythmias or myocardial infarction that can reduce the cerebral perfusion

Non-bedside investigations

- *Haematology*: the full blood count (FBC) needs to be assessed for presence of infection, e.g. leucocytosis, neutrophilia and anaemia

- *Biochemistry*: this includes serum electrolytes and base renal function (U&Es), e.g. sodium, potassium, calcium, phosphate and magnesium to correct electrolyte disturbances, and urea and creatinine to help guide fluid therapy. The inclusion of liver function tests (LFTs) helps to determine hypoalbuminaemia
- *Microbiology (sepsis screen)*: blood cultures, wound swabs, urine and sputum cultures to detect the presence of occult infection
- *Radiology*: such as a chest radiograph to detect a chest infection

What is the purpose of sedation in the critical care setting?
- Anxiolysis
- Analgesia
- Amnesia
- Hypnosis

Thus, there is a reduction in the level of consciousness, but retention of verbal communication. There is much variability on which permutations of these effects individual agents produce. Therefore, from a practical perspective in the intensive care setting, they are used to permit tolerance of endotracheal tubes, oral suction and other bedside procedures.

How is the level of sedation determined?
There are a number of techniques in routine clinical use to determine the level of sedation attained. The most commonly

employed of these is the Ramsay scoring system that describes six levels of sedation

- *Level 1 (awake)*: the patient is anxious and agitated or restless, or both
- *Level 2 (awake)*: the patient is cooperative, orientated and tranquil
- *Level 3 (awake)*: responds to commands only
- *Level 4 (asleep)*: brisk response to glabellar tap or loud auditory stimulus
- *Level 5 (asleep)*: sluggish response to glabellar tap or loud auditory stimulus
- *Level 6 (asleep)*: no response to glabellar tap or loud auditory stimulus

The ideally sedated patient attains levels 2–4.

Which classes of drugs may be used?

The most commonly used classes of drugs are

- *Benzodiazepines*: e.g. diazepam, midazolam and lorazepam, and may be administered as an oral or IV dose
- *Opiate analgesics*: morphine and the synthetic opioids, e.g. pethidine and fentanyl are popular choices. They may be combined effectively with benzodiazepines
- *Butyrophenones*: e.g. haloperidol, and as a group they are neurotransmitter-blocking drugs but require careful dosing in the elderly
- *Anaesthetic agents*: such as IV propofol and ketamine, and inhalational anaesthetic agents such as nitrous oxide (70%)

- *Trichloroethanol derivatives*: such as chloral hydrate
- *Phenothiazines*: e.g. chlorpromazine. They also act on neurotransmitter receptors

Which of these are the most commonly used for sedation in critical care?

The most commonly used sedative drugs on a Level 0–3 environment include benzodiazepines, opioid analgesics and butyrophenones. On a Level 3 environment the above classes of drug are used but anaesthetic agents, e.g. propofol, are also used.

What is the major physiological side effect of propofol?

Propofol can cause hypotension on induction, by decreasing the systemic vascular resistance, myocardial depression or both. As with many of the other sedatives, it also leads to respiratory depression.

Complex concepts

Brainstem death and organ donation

Which organs may be donated?

Organs

- Kidneys
- Heart
- Lungs
- Liver

- Pancreas
- Small bowel

Tissues

- Corneas
- Skin
- Bone and tendon
- Heart valves
- Cartilage

What are the general criteria that must be met prior to donation?

- Diagnosis of brainstem death, e.g. donation after brainstem death (DBD), and circulatory death, e.g. donation after circulatory death (DCD) must be established
- The donor is maintained on a ventilator in the absence of untreated sepsis
- There must not be a history of malignancy (primary brain tumours are exempt because of the confined nature of the disease)
- The donor must be HIV and HBV negative
- Those from high-risk groups, e.g. IV drug abusers, are excluded

There is some variation on these requirements depending on the organ to be donated, e.g. no history of myocardial infarction for heart donors and no history of alcohol abuse among liver donors. NB. Those with diabetes mellitus, smokers and those with HCV are not immediately excluded.

Which law governs organ donation in the UK?

There are currently two key laws governing organ donation and transplantation in the UK

- The Human Tissue (Scotland) Act 2006
- The Human Tissue Act 2004 (England, Wales and Northern Ireland)

Why is managing fluid balance particularly important when optimising the physiology of the organ donor?

Those with brainstem death develop cranial diabetes insipidus (DI) following loss of posterior pituitary function, leading to free water loss. This manifests as a large urine output (>4 ml/kg/h) and a co-existent rising plasma osmolality and hypernatraemia (Na^+ >145 mmol/L). It may be temporarily corrected using IV dextrose, but in severe cases, management requires an infusion of vasopressin to control the urine output. It occurs in 65%.

What other physiological changes may occur with brainstem death?

There are several reasons that contribute to rendering an organ not suitable for transplantation after DBD

- *Chronic disease*: obesity, hypertension and resultant end-organ damage, e.g. cardiac damage
- *Iatrogenic*: organ damage can be sustained due to adverse somatic consequences of brain-directed therapies
- *Pathological*: due to the pathophysiological consequences

Specific complications include

- *Hypotension*: occurs due to the loss of sympathetic peripheral vascular tone. This may require inotropic support of the mean arterial pressure (MAP) and organ perfusion. It occurs in 81%
- *Coagulopathy*: e.g. disseminated intravascular coagulation (DIC), may result from hypothermia and occurs in 28%
- *Hypothermia*: this occurs following the loss of thermo-regulation in the hypothalamus. This is exacerbated by reduced muscular and metabolic activity together with peripheral vasodilatation. It is managed by using surface heating blankets and warmed IV fluids (NB. hypothermia needs to be corrected before a diagnosis of brainstem death can be made correctly)
- *Hypertension (an initial finding)*: due to an immediate increase in sympathetic activity. This can lead to cardiovascular instability with arrhythmia formation in 28% of patients
- *Endocrine changes*: following loss of anterior pituitary function. The most important consequence is loss of thyroid hormone production leading to further arrhythmias (~28% of patients). The hormone tri-iodothyronine (T_3) may be administered as an infusion to help stabilise the patient in these situations

Other complications include neurogenic pulmonary oedema, which occurs in 18%, and, due to inadequate organ tissue

perfusion and oxygenation, metabolic acidosis can develop in
11% of patients.

How can donations after brainstem death be optimised physiologically?

Some basic steps include

- *Fluid balance*: this requires correction of hypovolaemia and
  diabetes insipidus
- *Drugs*: the introduction of vasopressin, weaning of inotropes
  and giving methylprednisolone (15 mg/kg) to attenuate the
  systemic inflammation of brainstem death
- *Ventilation*: recruitment manoeuvres to correct atelectasis
  that follows apnoea testing

Under which circumstances is it appropriate to perform an examination to confirm brainstem death?

Clinical evaluation of the patient for the diagnosis of brainstem
death must be justified, and so some preconditions must be
met

- *Coma*: this must be a deep coma and the patient must be
  reliant entirely on mechanical ventilation due to complete
  absence of spontaneous ventilation (apnoeic coma)
- *Brain damage*: which must be irreversible and compatible
  with a diagnosis of brainstem death

Those with the following potentially reversible causes of coma
should be identified and excluded

- *Drugs*: co-existent medications that could precipitate a crises and alcohol intoxication
- *Endocrine disturbances*: e.g. hypothyroidism, uraemic or hepatic encephalopathy
- *Metabolic disturbances*: e.g. hypoglycaemia or sodium imbalance
- *Hypothermia*: a core temperature of $<35°C$

What are the criteria for clinical confirmation of brainstem death?

The tests involve both an evaluation of the brainstem reflexes and the respiratory drive.

- No respiratory drive
  - *Progressive hypercarbia*: the subject is pre-oxygenated with 100% oxygen and then disconnected from the ventilator for 10 minutes while the $PaCO_2$ is permitted to rise. Normally, respiration is stimulated above a $PaCO_2$ of 6.65 kPa
- No brainstem function
  - Absent pupillary light reflex (CN II, III)
  - Absent corneal reflex (CN V, VII)
  - Absent cranial nerve motor function (CN V, VII)
  - Absent gag and cough reflex following pharyngeal and bronchial stimulation with a suction catheter (CN IX)
  - Absent vestibulo-ocular test following a cold caloric test (CN VIII, III)

The test should be repeated to decrease observer bias after an unspecified length of time for full confirmation.

Who may legally perform these tests?

The test must be performed by two clinicians who work in relevant areas of expertise, e.g. intensive care, anaesthesia, neurology or neurosurgery. One of them should be a consultant and the other must have been registered with the General Medical Council (GMC) for at least 5 years. They should not be part of the transplant team.

Under which clinical circumstances can confirmation prove difficult?

- Chronic obstructive pulmonary disease
- Eye injuries or pre-existing eye disease
- Brainstem encephalitis

Circulatory support: inotropic agents

In which ways may the failing cardiovascular system be supported?

The cardiovascular system may need support if there is a fall in the cardiac index to below 2.2 L/min/m^2 or in the situation of septic shock when peripheral circulatory failure results in a fall in the systemic vascular resistance (SVR) and arterial pressure. It may be supported by the following means

- Inotropic agents
- Chronotropic drugs and cardiac pacing
- Vasoconstrictors
- Vasodilators

- Mechanical, e.g. intra-arterial balloon pump counter-pulsation (IABP), extracorporeal membrane oxygenation (ECMO), ventricular-assist device (VAD)

Give some examples of commonly used drugs for this purpose

- Catecholamines
  - *Adrenergic agonists*: adrenaline, noradrenaline, isoprenaline increase the systemic vascular resistance (SVR) through vasoconstriction, heart rate, stroke volume and resultant cardiac output to increase the systolic blood pressure
  - *Dopaminergic agents (with some adrenergic activity)*: dopamine, dobutamine, dopexamine increase the heart rate, stroke volume and resultant cardiac output and contractility to increase the blood pressure, but depending on dose, decrease the SVR to produce vasodilatation
- Non-catecholamines
  - *Phosphodiesterase III (PDE III) inhibitors*: milrinone, enoximone increase the contractility, stroke volume but decrease SVR by vasodilatation (so-called inodilators)
  - *Calcium channel agonists*: levosimendan, calcium chloride produces a transient inotropic effect. They increase the sensitivity of myocardial troponin to intracellular calcium
  - *ADH agonist*: vasopressin is the natural analogue and increases systemic vascular resistance through vasoconstriction to increase arterial pressure

Draw a table comparing the effects of the different inotropes on adrenergic receptors

Table 6.1

Drug	α_1	β_1	β_2	DA_1	Dose (μg/kg/min)
Dopamine					
Low dose				+++	1–4
Medium dose			+	+++	5–10
High dose	+		+	+++	>10

Comments

Dose-dependent effects. Increased splanchnic/renal blood flow and diuretic effect at low doses, but no evidence for renal protective activity. May inhibit gastric emptying

Drug	α_1	β_1	β_2	DA_1	Dose
Dopexamine	0	0	+++	++	0.5–6.0

Comments

Inodilator licensed for treatment of heart failure following cardiac surgery. Increases hepatosplanchnic blood flow, and may ameliorate gut ischaemia in SIRS

Drug	α_1	β_1	β_2	DA_1	Dose
Dobutamine	0	+++	++	0	2.5–10.0

Comments

Inodilator, useful in low output/high systemic vascular resistance (SVR) states such as cardiogenic shock
Unlikely to be of benefit in the hypotension associated with sepsis/SIRS

Drug	α_1	β_1	β_2	DA_1	Dose
Salbutamol	0	+	+++	0	0.1–1.0

Comments

Useful in treatment of acute severe asthma

Drug	α_1	β_1	β_2	DA_1	Dose
Adrenaline	+++	+++	++	0	0.01–0.20

(*cont.*)

Drug	α_1	β_1	β_2	DA_1	Dose (μg/kg/min)

Comments

Useful first-line inotrope. High β-adrenoceptor activity, increasing cardiac output. Vasodilatation may be seen at low doses, vasoconstriction at higher doses

| **Noradrenaline** | +++ | + | 0 | 0 | 0.01–0.20 |

Comments

Inoconstrictor. Very useful in high output/low SVR states such as severe SIRS/sepsis. Inotropic effect via myocardial α-receptors and β-activity. May cause reflex bradycardia. Risk of peripheral and splanchnic ischaemia

| **Isoprenaline** | 0 | +++ | +++ | 0 | 0.01–0.20 |

Comments

Potent β-agonist, hence risk of tachydysrhythmias. Generally reserved for emergency treatment of bradydysrhythmias and AV block prior to pacing. Now replaced by salbutamol in the management of acute severe asthma

| **Phenylephrine** | +++ | 0 | 0 | 0 | 0.2–1.0 |

Comments

Pure vasoconstrictor. Useful alternative to noradrenaline (e.g. if arrhythmias are a problem)

The underlying effect is dependent on dose and rate of administration, e.g. in dopamine (*see* below).

Elaborate on the mechanism of action of the phosphodiesterase inhibitors (PDE III)

The PDE III inhibitors act by inhibiting the hydrolysis and degradation of intracellular cyclic AMP (cAMP). This causes an increase in the intracellular concentration of calcium ions, leading to enhanced cardiac contractility and stroke volume.

What is the effect of PDE III on cardiovascular function?

These agents improve cardiac output by two important mechanisms

- *Afterload reduction*: reduction of systemic and pulmonary vascular resistance decreases the afterload. This is particularly useful in the situation of cardiogenic shock associated with a high systemic vascular resistance. Also useful in cases of right ventricular dysfunction with pulmonary hypertension
- *Inotropic enhancement*: there is an increase in the heart rate but decreased myocardial oxygen due to a lowering of filling pressures

Before inotropes are commenced, what safeguards must be in place?

Prior to using inotropes, adequate cardiovascular monitoring should be in place (*see* Chapter 3, Cardiac Assessment). The minimum includes the presence of continuous pulse oximetry, arterial line, and central venous pressure catheter, ECG monitoring and urethral catheterisation.

What are the effects of dopamine on the circulation?

- *Low doses (1–3 µg/kg/min)*: dopamine acts on dopaminergic receptors
- *Medium doses (1–3 µg/kg/min)*: it acts on β1-receptors. At higher doses (>10–15 µg/kg/min) it acts on β1-receptors and α1-receptors. Thus, at medium doses, it causes renal vasodilatation, increasing renal perfusion to cause diuresis

and natriuresis. However, evidence suggests that some of the improved urine output is due to a direct inotropic effect

- *Higher doses*: it causes vasoconstriction, to increase afterload and peripheral resistance and mean arterial pressure. One risk of using dopamine are tachyarrhythmias

What are the indications for use of noradrenaline?

Noradrenaline, having mainly $\alpha1$-effects, is a potent vasoconstrictor that is useful in supporting the arterial pressure in cases of septic shock. The resulting vasoconstriction leads to reduced peripheral perfusion, e.g. decreased renal perfusion, and increased afterload that reduces stroke volume and increases myocardial oxygen demand at high doses despite improved arterial pressure. It can also be used with PDE III inhibitors, so that the patient benefits from an increased ejection fraction, without excessive vasodilatation.

What are the effects of adrenaline on the circulation?

- At low doses towards the bottom of the range (0.01–0.15 μg/kg/min), the $\beta1$-effects predominate
- At higher doses towards the top of the range (0.01–0.15 μg/kg/min), the $\alpha1$-effects predominate.

Therefore, at low doses it increases the cardiac output and reduces the SVR. Conversely, at higher doses, there is an increase in the afterload and arterial pressure due to increases in the SVR. Although providing increased coronary blood flow, it also can increase the myocardial oxygen demand. It also causes lactic acidosis, even at low doses.

What about dobutamine?

Having strong $\beta1$-effects, it has both inotropic and chronotropic effects, increasing the cardiac output. However, it also can reduce the systemic vascular resistance through $\beta2$-stimulation, potentially leading to reduced blood pressure. It is useful in situations where the cardiac output is low with increased SVR.

What are the general problems associated with the use of inotropes?

Some of the problems of inotropic agents are:

- Tachyarryhythmias
- Bradycardia, e.g. noradrenaline
- Hypertension, e.g. adrenaline
- Hypotension, e.g. dobutamine, PDE III inhibitors

Despite being essential to maintain blood pressure, inotropes increase myocardial oxygen consumption and demand, placing an additional strain on myocardial function.

What can be done if the cardiac index is still poor despite maximum inotrope use?

In these situations the circulation can be supported by using an intra-aortic balloon pump, which can be inserted in the ICU setting.

How does an intra-aortic balloon pump work?

The basic principle involves mechanical assistance to the failing heart through afterload reduction and an improvement of the coronary blood flow. The device sits in the descending aorta and is connected to an external console that pumps helium in and out of the balloon in phase with the ECG. The balloon expands in diastole causing an increase in the coronary perfusion pressure. By deflating just before the onset of systole, it leads to afterload reduction, reducing impedance to left ventricular ejection and reduced myocardial demand. It is thrombogenic, so anticoagulation is required.

How and where is an intra-aortic balloon inserted?

It may be inserted at the time of cardiac surgery or in the ICU through the femoral artery at the groin, using the Seldinger technique.

Endotracheal intubation

How may the trachea be intubated, and which routes are used?

The tracheal should only be intubated by healthcare professional trained in advanced airway techniques, e.g. an anaesthetist, and two routes are generally used, orotracheal and nasotracheal.

What are the indications for intubation?

Indications include

Operative

- *Endotracheal*: standard anaesthesia when using IPPV and muscle relaxation for most general anaesthetic surgical procedures

- *Endobronchial*: dual lumen endobronchial tube to permit one lung ventilation during thoracic, cardiac and oesophagogastric surgical procedures

Non-operative

- *Airway protection*: from gastric contents which may be aspirated, e.g. in cases of severe head injury when ventilation is also required, and to permit airway suction
- *Cardiorespiratory resuscitation (CPR)*: to provide a definitive airway and rule out one of the reversible causes, e.g. hypoxia during the ALS algorithm

Remember, once a patient is intubated outside the context of undergoing an operation, in a hospital setting, you automatically escalate their treatment of care to that of ICU.

What are the basic steps involved in intubation under general anaesthesia?

- *Pre-oxygenation*: where 100% oxygen is administered for 3–5 minutes
- *Positioning*: the neck is extended
- *Anaesthesia*: the type is administered depending on the indication, e.g. local for awake intubation or general
- *Muscle relaxation*: this is used if a general anaesthetic is being administered
- *Intubation*: this occurs in sequential steps, laryngoscopy, and intubation, cuff inflation using air and connection of the tube to an oxygen source. A bougie can be used as a guide wire over which the tube is sited

- *Auscultation*: checks correct position, e.g. audible breath sounds in one lung could mean inadvertent endobronchial intubation, so pull back the tube
- *Security*: the tube is taped in place using cotton tape

What is the purpose of pre-oxygenation prior to intubation?

The purpose is to delay the time before hypoxaemia occurs during intubation by increasing the PaO_2.

What is the difference between a Magill and Macintosh laryngoscope?

The Magill is a straight-bladed instrument, and the Macintosh has a curved blade.

What shape of laryngoscope blade is used for paediatric anaesthesia and why?

A straight-bladed laryngoscope is used for paediatric intubation. In children, the epiglottis is floppy and U-shaped. The straight blade passes behind the epiglottis, fixing it in position, so that it can be lifted forward to expose the laryngeal opening.

What common sizes of laryngeal tube are available for the adult?

Common sizes are 8.0 mm in males and 7.0 mm in females (the size refers to the internal diameter).

Is a general anaesthetic always required for intubation?

No, awake intubation is achieved with a local-anaesthetic throat spray or nerve block. It is performed in those at risk of imminent airway obstruction if a general anaesthetic and muscle relaxation is used.

What is rapid sequence induction, and what important features define this form of intubation?

This is required for emergency induction of anaesthesia, e.g. ruptured abdominal aortic aneurysm (rAAA), where there is a risk of gastric aspiration. The important requirements are a skilled assistant, suction equipment at the ready and cricoid pressure applied by the assistant. This pressure is released only when the cuff is inflated. Traditionally, IV suxamethonium is used to achieve rapid muscle relaxation.

When is nasotracheal intubation performed?

- Head and neck procedures, e.g. ENT, Max-Fax and neurosurgery

It can be considered when long-term intubation is anticipated, since there is no interference with the mouth.

What are the complications of endotracheal intubation?

- *Trauma*: to the upper airway structures, e.g. teeth, pharynx and larynx can all get damaged
- *Spinal injury*: to those with an unstable neck, e.g. trauma, rheumatoid neck
- *Acute hypertension*: upon laryngoscopy due to an autonomic reflex
- *Spasm*: laryngospasm, or bronchospasm, can be life-threatening

- *Misplacement*: this can occur due to inadvertent bronchial intubation, oesophageal intubation
- *Disconnection*: inadvertent extubation or disconnection from the gas supply

Ultimately, mucosal ulceration and tracheal stenosis can occur if long-term use is deemed necessary, and gastric aspiration is always a potential possibility.

How long can a tube be left in place?

Generally, the tube is not left for more than 2 weeks, to prevent long-term complications. A tracheostomy may be performed if prolonged intubation is anticipated.

Extubation and weaning

What are some of the prerequisites to successful extubation?

The original disease process that leads to the requirement for ventilation must be resolved. Other requirements include

- *Respiratory*: adequate lung function
- *Cardiovascular*: haemodynamic stability
- *Gastrointestinal*: nutrition must be satisfactory
- *Neurological*: the GCS should be adequate, e.g. must be good enough to obey commands. So there should be no confusion or agitation that may jeopardise success. This requires a progressive reversal of sedation
- *General*: no sign of sepsis as this increases the metabolic and respiratory demands, as well as increasing CO_2 production

What is meant by 'adequate' lung function in this context?

Some satisfactory lung function parameters are

- Respiratory rate <35/min
- PaO_2 >11 kPa (FiO_2 of <0.5)
- Minute volume <10 L/min
- Vital capacity >10 ml/kg
- Tidal volume >5 ml/kg
- Maximum inspiratory force >20 cmH$_2$O

These parameters can vary depending on the underlying indication for intubation, the disease process, progress and eventual anticipated outcome.

Why should nutrition be optimised prior to extubating the chronically ventilated?

There are two main reasons

- *Increases muscle strength*: the nutritional state affects respiratory muscle strength and fatigability
- *Reduces CO_2 production*: excess reliance on glucose as the major source of carbohydrate leads to increased CO_2 production. This may lead to increased ventilator demands, and so failure to wean

Briefly mention some of the ventilation strategies used to wean from mechanical ventilation

- *T-piece ventilation*: added to the end of the circuit, and can be used just prior to extubation. When used on its own, it is more successful in those who have been intubated for a short period of time only (a couple of days at the maximum)

- *T-piece and CPAP*: one of the problems of intubation is that it abolishes the small amount of natural PEEP provided by the laryngeal complex. The use of CPAP enhances the residual PEEP, permitting the T-piece to be used for longer periods in those who require it. Thus, during weaning, the T-piece is left on during parts of the day, while mechanical ventilation is continued at night
- *Intermittent mandatory ventilation (IMV)*: the ventilator provides a certain tidal volume at a specified rate. Between these mechanical breaths, the patient supplements with their own, spontaneous breaths. The mandatory rate is progressively reduced, while increasing the spontaneous breaths
- *Pressure support ventilation*: the patient breathes spontaneously, but each breath is augmented with a positive inspiratory pressure. This is progressively reduced until full extubation or CPAP

ICU admission criteria

What are the levels of intensity of care of hospital patients?
Care of hospital patients according to The Intensive Care Society may be divided into four levels

- *Level 0*: the ward environment meeting the needs of the patient in an acute hospital
- *Level 1*: the ward patient requires the input of the critical care team for advice on optimisation of care in an acute setting

- *Level 2*: high dependency unit (HDU) care includes more detailed observation and intervention, often for a single failing organ system or post-operative care following major surgery
- *Level 3*: intensive care unit (ICU) care for the support and management of two or more failing systems or for advanced respiratory support

What is the purpose of the intensive care unit?

The intensive care unit provides advanced respiratory, cardiovascular and renal monitoring and support. It follows that conditions requiring support and monitoring must be thought reversible at the time of admission to the unit.

Give some criteria for admitting patients to the ICU

- *Respiratory*: advanced respiratory support is required, i.e. intubation and mechanical ventilation
- *System support*: two or more organs need to be supported, e.g. respiratory and renal failure
- *Reversibility*: the disease process is considered to be reversible as ICU is not the place to palliate patients

NB. There is a legal duty to uphold the wishes of the patient regarding their ceiling of care, e.g. advanced directives.

How does the cost of ICU care compare to ordinary ward care?

It has been estimated that ICU care is some 3–4 times more expensive than routine ward care.

What other departments must be found in the vicinity of the ICU?

- Accident & Emergency
- Operating rooms/Catheter labs
- Radiology

Mechanical ventilation and support

Give some basic indications for the use of invasive ventilatory support

The basic effects of mechanical ventilation are improved oxygenation and carbon dioxide elimination. Some of the indications are

- Respiratory rate >35/min, with imminent exhaustion
- Tidal volume <5 ml/kg
- Vital capacity <10–15 ml/kg
- PaO_2 <8 kPa (FiO_2 of >0.6), e.g. inadequate oxygenation despite sustained attempts to oxygenate
- $PaCO_2$ >8 kPa, e.g. inadequate ventilation, due to exhaustion
- ICP >20 mmHg: keeping the $PaCO_2$ ~4.0–4.5 kPa promotes cerebral vasoconstriction, and, hence, reduces the intracranial pressure. This may occur at the expense of reducing oxygenation

Note that the use of ventilation must be appropriate given the prognosis of the disease, and these values can vary depending on the clinical context.

Which parameters of ventilation may be adjusted on the mechanical ventilator?

Some parameters that may be adjusted (depending on the type of ventilator used) are

- *Respiratory rate*: the normal range is 12–16/min
- *Tidal volume*: 5–7 ml/kg
- *Fraction of inspired oxygen (FiO$_2$)*: 0.21–1.0
- *Flow waveform*: a sinusoidal flow during the respiratory cycle reduces the mean airway pressures
- *Inspiratory:expiratory (I:E) ratio*: usually 1:2
- *Pressure limit*: to prevent barotraumas and iatrogenic pneumothoraces
- *PEEP and CPAP*: the addition of these components delivers additional pressure at the end of the cycle

Which parameters need to be adjusted to improve oxygenation?

- ↑FiO$_2$
- ↑PEEP
- ↑I:E ratio, e.g. the length of the inspiratory phase is increased

Which parameters need to be adjusted to improve ventilation?

Ventilation (the ability to 'blow off' CO$_2$) may be improved by

- ↑respiratory rate
- ↑tidal volume
- ↑peak pressure

What are the basic modes of ventilation?

- *Pressure control*: either a pre-set inspiratory pressure is delivered, or the cycle changes from inspiration to expiration when a certain pressure is reached
- *Volume control*: a fixed tidal volume is delivered, and is generally used by older and simpler circuits
- *Assisted modes*: the ventilator augments each inspiratory effort initiated by the patient, either by pressure or volume support, e.g. pressure support ventilation (PSV), synchronised intermittent mandatory ventilation (SIMV)

What is positive end-expiratory pressure (PEEP) and what physiological changes occur with it?

PEEP is used in conjunction with IPPV and involves delivery of additional pressure (5–20 cmH$_2$O) at the end of the respiratory cycle to prevent alveolar collapse at the end of expiration. Thus, oxygenation is improved when additional alveoli are recruited. Other than alveolar recruitment, some of the other physiological effects are

- ↑Compliance
- ↑Functional residual capacity (FRC), and this increases the compliance
- ↓Physiological shunting increases the V/Q ratio

Give some examples of the physiological effects and complications of intermittent positive pressure ventilation (IPPV)

- *Respiratory*: over-distension of the lungs produces barotrauma in the form of alveolar rupture. This manifests

predominantly as pneumothorax or pneumomediastinum.
Also increases the risk of nosocomial pneumonia

- *Cardiovascular*: by making the intrathoracic pressure less
  negative, it reduces the venous return to the heart. The lung
  expansion also distorts alveolar capillaries, increasing the
  pulmonary vascular resistance. These have the effect of
  reducing the cardiac output and arterial pressure. Therefore,
  tissue oxygen delivery may be impaired
- *Renal*: leads to a reduction of the renal perfusion pressure,
  and hence the urine output
- *Paralytic ileus*: caused by uncertain mechanisms, but more
  probably associated to co-existing infective and
  inflammatory conditions

Pulmonary artery catheters

Define the cardiac output
The cardiac output (CO) equals the heart rate (HR) multiplied
by the stroke volume (SV). It is ∼5–6 L/min

$$CO = HR \times SV$$

Define the cardiac index
The cardiac index (CI) is the cardiac output divided by the
body surface area (BSA). The minimum acceptable level for
adequate tissue perfusion is 2.2–2.5 L/min/m^2.

What is a pulmonary artery catheter and what purpose does it serve?
This is a multi-lumen, balloon-tipped, flow-directed catheter
that is passed through the right heart and into the pulmonary

artery. It provides a more useful picture of left heart function other than CVP measures alone, and can be used to calculate a number of useful parameters of cardiovascular function in the critically ill, thus providing both severity assessment and therapeutic guidance.

By which principle does it reflect left heart function?
When it is wedged in a branch of the pulmonary artery, i.e. the balloon is inflated in a branch of the PA, there is a continuous column of blood beyond the tip of the catheter that extends to the left atrium. Therefore, the pulmonary artery pressure at the wedged position is equal to the left atrial pressure. This is called the pulmonary artery capillary wedge pressure (PACWP).

Give some indications for its use
The indications for its use are controversial, variable and not absolute

- *Drugs*: concomitant with the use of inotropic support, especially vasodilators
- *Surgical*: post-cardiac surgery in those with poor left ventricular function and pulmonary hypertension
- *Respiratory*: those with suspected ARDS and pulmonary oedema
- *Cardiovascular*: shock of any cause
- Those with multi-organ failure and multiple injuries with a thoracic component

What physiological parameters does it measure directly?
- Mean arterial pressure (MAP)

- Heart rate (HR)
- Mean pulmonary artery pressure (MPAP)
- Cardiac output (CO)
- Pulmonary artery capillary wedge pressure (PACWP)
- Ejection fraction (EF)
- Mixed venous oxygen saturation (SvO_2)

What are the derived variables?

- Cardiac index (CI)
- Stroke volume (SV)
- Systemic vascular resistance (SVR)
- Pulmonary vascular resistance (PVR)
- Indexed SVR and PVR (these values divided by the Body Surface Area)
- Oxygen delivery and oxygen consumption

Define the systemic vascular resistance

The systemic vascular resistance $= \dfrac{MAP - CVP}{CO} \times 80$.

The normal range is 900–1400 dyn/s/cm^{-5}.

Define the pulmonary vascular resistance

The pulmonary vascular resistance $= \dfrac{MPAP - PAOP}{CO} \times 80$.

The normal range is 150–250 dyn/s/cm^{-5}.

What are the complications of insertion?

These include complications from central line insertion (*see* Central Access: Central Lines)

- *Cardiac arrhythmias*: most commonly atrial and ventricular ectopics. Ventricular tachycardia and ventricular fibrillation as well as heart block also reported
- *Cardiac valve injury*: leading to incompetence of the tricuspid or pulmonary valves
- *Pulmonary artery rupture*: presents as shock and haemoptysis and occurs from injury by the J-wire or following balloon inflation
- *Pulmonary infarction*: if the balloon is kept in the wedged position for too long. Also occurs if there is embolisation of a thrombus formed at the catheter tip or catheter migration

Other complications include the catheter knotting and generalised sepsis from the presence of a foreign body. Therefore, it requires some expertise and an aseptic non-touch sterile technique for insertion.

By which principle is the cardiac output measured?
The cardiac output is measured using the indicator dilution or the thermodilution techniques. Both of these have similar principles. With the indicator dilution technique, indocyanine green is injected into the circulation and samples are taken peripherally from the radial artery. A graph of the concentration of the dye in the peripheral blood over time is plotted. The cardiac output equates to the amount of dye injected divided by the area under the curve.

In the case of the thermodilution method, 10 ml of cold crystalloid is injected peripherally, and the change of temperature detected by a thermistor at the end of the catheter. A graph is also plotted for the change of temperature

of the blood passing the thermistor against time. This graph is
used to calculate the cardiac output.

Renal replacement therapy

What types of renal replacement therapies are available?
These may be continuous or intermittent therapies

- *Haemodialysis*: continuous or intermittent
- *Haemofiltration*: a continuous form of renal replacement
- *Combination of dialysis and filtration*: continuous
  haemodiafiltration
- *Peritoneal dialysis*: continuous or intermittent

What are the indications for commencing these?
The agreed indications for replacement therapy in acute
kidney injury or chronic kidney disease are

- Refractory fluid overload
- Hyperkalaemia of >6.5 mmol/L
- Acidosis of pH <7.1
- Urea >30 mmol/L
- Creatinine >300 μmol/L
- Uraemic complications, e.g. encephalopathy, pericarditis,
  neuropathy or myopathy
- Drug overdose

**What are the basic features of haemodialysis
and haemofiltration?**
- *Haemodialysis*: the principle is that the blood interfaces the
  dialysis solution across a selectively permeable membrane

which permits the passage of molecules of <5 kDa down a diffusion gradient. Unlike haemofiltration, it may be administered as either an intermittent or a continuous regimen

- *Haemofiltration*: this relies on the continuous convection of molecules across a membrane to which they are permeable. The fluid that is removed from the patient is replaced with a buffered physiological solution. Thus it is more effective in removing large volumes of fluid, but is not as effective as dialysis in clearing smaller molecules

When is intermittent haemodialysis used, and what are the basic components of the circuit?

This may be used several times per week in those with chronic kidney disease and much less commonly used in the critically ill patient with acute kidney injury. The essential components of the circuit are

- *Vascular access*: which may be through a central line or a surgical arteriovenous fistula for use in the long term
- *Extracorporeal circuit*: this has an air trap and heparin pump to prevent air emboli and clotting in the circuit, respectively
- *Dialysis machine*: the dialysate solution passes through a dialyser cartridge that houses the diffusion membrane. Blood passes through and permits diffusion across to the dialysate at the membrane interface

The circuit is driven by a roller pump.

Give the most important complications of haemodialysis

- *Dysequilibrium syndrome*: this follows sudden changes in the serum osmolality that occurs when molecules such as urea are filtered out. It can lead to cerebral oedema that usually presents with headaches, nausea and occasionally seizures
- *Hypotension*: following a sudden reduction in the intravascular volume
- *Immune reactions*: may occur when the extracorporeal circuit causes systemic complement cascade activation
- *Hypoxia*: as part of the systemic immune response leading to neutrophil aggregation in the lungs
- *Sepsis*: from the indwelling line
- Loss of circuit connection leading to air embolism or haemorrhage

What types of continuous renal replacement therapies are there?

There are a number of continuous renal replacement modalities, depending on whether they rely on dialysis or filtration, and on the pattern of vascular connection

- *Continuous arteriovenous haemofiltration (CAVH)*: the flow is driven by the arteriovenous pressure difference
- *Continuous venovenous haemofiltration (CVVH)*: flow relies on roller pumps and so does not depend on the unstable arterial pressure of the critically ill patient (NB. good vascular access is required)

- *Continuous arteriovenous or venovenous haemodialysis (CAVHD/CVVHD)*: this is useful for slow ultrafiltration and diffusion of solutes, and the solution runs countercurrent to the direction of blood
- *Continuous arteriovenous or venovenous haemodiafiltration (CAVHDF/CVVHDF)*: a combination of both techniques that provides the best rate of urea clearance and is useful for hypercatabolic patients

How does peritoneal dialysis work?

Peritoneal dialysis is a slow form of continuous dialysis that relies on the peritoneum and its capillary network to act as the selectively permeable membrane. As with haemodialysis, solute flows down a diffusion gradient, and fluid flows by osmosis. The dialysate is introduced into the peritoneum by way of a Tenckhoff catheter and dwells within the abdomen for several hours before being drained off.

This technique has been used in the intensive care setting, but has been superseded by other replacement therapies that are faster and more effective in removing urea and other solutes. However, it still has a place in the haemodynamically unstable patient and the ambulating patient with chronic renal failure.

It is particularly useful in the paediatric setting when vascular access can be difficult.

What is the classical infective complication? How is this recognised and treated?

The important infective complication is peritonitis that occurs following introduction of exogenous organisms. It may initially be recognised by the presence of a turbid effluent when the dialysate is drained, with >50 white cells per ml. It is caused by gram-positive organisms in 75% of cases, predominantly *Staphylococcus epidermidis* and *Staphylococcus aureus*. Occasionally it is fungal. It may be managed by the addition of broad spectrum antibiotics to the dialysate, such as cefuroxime and gentamicin.

Septic shock and multi-organ dysfunction syndrome (MODS)

What is an endotoxin?

An endotoxin is composed of lipopolysaccharides derived from the cell walls of gram-negative bacteria, and is the most common causative agent of septic shock. It has three components

- Lipid A, e.g. the lipid portion, and is the source of much of the molecule's systemic effects
- Core polysaccharide
- Oligosaccharide side chains

What is the difference between bacteraemia, sepsis and severe sepsis?

- *Bacteraemia*: the presence of viable bacteria in the circulation
- *Sepsis*: the syndrome associated with the systemic response to infection, e.g. presence of >2 SIRS criteria due to infection. It is characterised by a systemic inflammatory response and diffuse tissue injury

- *Severe sepsis*: this is sepsis with organ dysfunction, hypoperfusion and hypotension (systolic <90 mmHg), e.g. lactic acidosis, decreased urine output and altered GCS

NB. Infection is a process (abnormal presence of microbes), sepsis is the syndrome resulting from the host's immune response.

Define septic shock

This is the presence of sepsis associated with hypotension (systolic BP <90 mmHg) or hypoperfusion resulting in organ dysfunction despite adequate fluid resuscitation (or the requirement for inotropes), e.g. persisting lactic acidosis, decreased urine output and altered GCS.

What particular feature distinguishes septic shock from cardiogenic or hypovolaemic shock?

The important feature of septic shock is the presence of a reduced systemic vascular resistance and increased cardiac output.

It has also been described as a distributive type of shock (*see* Chapter 3, Haemorrhagic Shock). The patient has warm and vasodilated peripheries. Cardiogenic or hypovolaemic shock is characterised by an increase in the systemic vascular resistance in response to a fall in the cardiac output. This manifests as cool peripheries reflecting the reduced cardiac index.

What is the systemic inflammatory response syndrome (SIRS)?

The systemic inflammatory response syndrome (SIRS) is the syndrome arising from the body's reaction to critical illness, e.g. overwhelming infection or trauma. Its presence is recognised and defined according to a number of clinical criteria

- Temperature of $>38°C$ or $<36°C$
- Heart rate of >90 bpm
- Respiratory rate $>20/min$ or PaCO$_2$ <4.3 kPa (<32 mmHg)
- White cell count $>12 \times 10^9$ or $<4 \times 10^9$ or $>10\%$ immature forms

What triggers SIRS?

Some triggers include

- Sepsis
- Multiple trauma
- Burns
- Acute pancreatitis

Thus many conditions other than sepsis may trigger these features. The concept of SIRS was introduced after it was shown that less than 50% of those who exhibited features of sepsis had positive blood cultures.

What are the basic pathophysiological events that lead to the development of SIRS?

The pathophysiology of this condition involves a progressive increase in the distribution of the inflammatory response in the body. The basic problem is a situation where the inflammatory response to the triggering event is excessive or poorly regulated. It has been described in terms of three phases

- *Phase I*: there is a local acute inflammatory response with the chemotaxis of neutrophil polymorphs and macrophages.

Inflammatory mediators such as cytokines and proteases are released

- *Phase II*: these mediators are systemically distributed. Normally anti-inflammatory mediators such as IL-10 ensure that the systemic response is limited
- *Phase III*: an overwhelming systemic cytokine storm leads to the recognised systemic outcomes, e.g. pyrexia, tachycardia, peripheral vasodilatation and increased vascular permeability. There is a catabolic state with reduced tissue oxygen delivery despite increased oxygen demand

Name some important mediators that have been implicated in the development of SIRS

- *IL-1*: induces pyrexia and leucocyte activation
- *IL-6*: involved in the acute phase response
- *IL-8*: involved in neutrophil chemotaxis
- *Platelet-activating factor (PAF)*: induces leucocyte activation and increased capillary permeability
- *Tumour necrosis factor alpha (TNF-α)*: a pyrogen that stimulates leucocytes

Have you heard of the 'two-hit' hypothesis in the development of SIRS?

Yes, this is the observed finding that those with SIRS who are recovering can have a rapid systemic response to a seemingly trivial second insult, e.g. a urinary tract or line infection. This may lead to a rapid and terminal deterioration in the patient's state.

Define the multi-organ dysfunction syndrome (MODS)

MODS is defined as the presence of altered, and potentially reversible, organ function in an acutely ill patient such that homeostasis cannot be maintained without intervention. By definition it affects two or more organs. There are two types

- *Primary MODS*: the organ failure is directly attributable to the initial insult, e.g. respiratory failure in pneumonia
- *Secondary MODS*: the failure occurs as a result of the effects of SIRS, e.g. acute kidney injury (AKI) secondary to septic shock. There may be a latent period between the initial event and the subsequent organ failure

Which organ systems may be involved in this process?

Any organ system may potentially be involved

- *Cardiovascular*: there is vasodilatation with microcirculatory changes that increase the capillary permeability. This leads to a reduction of the systemic vascular resistance and mal-distribution of blood flow. Initially, there is a hyperdynamic state with increased cardiac output. Later, there is myocardial impairment
- *Respiratory*: there is acute lung injury progressing to ARDS. This presents as pulmonary oedema leading to V/Q mismatch and respiratory failure
- *Renal*: this is manifested as acute kidney injury due to acute tubular necrosis
- *Gastrointestinal*: there is an ileus and intolerance to enteral feeding. Translocation of bacteria across a permeable gut

wall perpetuates sepsis. There can be deranged liver function leading to encephalopathy

- *Coagulopathy*: this is due to systemic activation of the coagulation cascade and can lead to disseminated intravascular coagulation
- *Others*: such as bone marrow failure and neurological disturbances

Why may the gut fail in these situations?

There are a number of reasons

- The mucosa is very sensitive to ischaemia and loses its integrity and function
- This is exacerbated by mal-distribution of blood flow
- There is an alteration in the number and type of gut flora

What is the mortality associated with organ failure?

In an intensive care environment

- Renal failure is around 20%
- Renal failure and one other organ is around 70%
- Renal failure and three failing organs is around 95%

What are the basic principles of management of any case of SIRS and MODS?

Management place a heavy emphasis on support of the failing organ systems

- *Surgical intervention*: sometimes required to reduce the infective load into the circulation, e.g. incision and drainage of pus
- *Circulatory support*: to maintain the cardiac index and oxygen delivery to the tissues, use IV fluids, e.g. colloids such

as red cells and crystalloids such as 0.9% saline. Inotropes may be required to increase the systemic vascular resistance (*see* Circulatory Support: Inotropic Agents). Monitoring therefore involves the insertion of a pulmonary artery flotation catheter

- *Respiratory support*: non-invasive or invasive ventilation may be required for the management of ARDS and respiratory failure. (NB. the risk of nosocomial pneumonia from intubation or aspiration)
- *Renal support*: to ensure that the urine output is >0.5 ml/kg/h. Dopamine or a furosemide infusion may be required to support the failing kidney. Cardiac support helps maintain the renal perfusion pressure. Renal replacement therapies may also be required
- *Nutritional support*: may be enteral or parenteral. Enteral nutrition helps maintain mucosal integrity and reduce bacterial translocation

During the early phases there is empirical use of broad spectrum antibiotics and surveillance of infection, but in the latter stages, agents are targeted to grown microbiological sensitivities from general, e.g. blood, and local, e.g. sputum, sources.

Transfer of the critically ill patient

What is meant by primary and secondary transfer?

- *Primary transfer*: is the movement of the patient from the scene of trauma to the site of hospital care. It is managed and organised by the pre-hospital team that usually comprises paramedics

- *Secondary transfer*: involves the movement of the patient
  between hospitals where they can receive specialist
  investigations and treatments, e.g. neurosurgical units for
  evacuation of an extradural haematoma

What types of transportation may be used to transfer the critically ill?

The principle forms of transport employed are

- *Ground ambulance*: providing door-to-door transport,
  but at the cost of reduced speed, e.g. commonly used in
  cities
- *Air ambulance*: either as a helicopter or aeroplane, but may
  include the added hazard of transfer at high altitude, e.g.
  commonly used in the highlands of Scotland

What are the dangers of a high altitude transfer?

There are two main dangers

- *Hypoxia*: due to a reduction in the atmospheric pressure
  associated with an increasing altitude. This is not usually a
  problem since the critically ill should receive supplemental
  oxygen from a cylinder
- *Gaseous expansion*: this leads to rapid tension of a simple
  pneumothorax if it goes unrecognised. For this reason,
  bilateral chest drains may be required prior to transfer in
  those with suspected chest injuries. It can also lead to
  worsening bowel distension in those with bowel
  obstruction

Which four groups of people are the most important as far as communication is concerned?

The four most important groups of people that need to be communicated with closely are

- The person who is to be transferred (if they are conscious)
- The transferring team, e.g. including the aircrew
- The receiving team
- The relatives of the patient (even if they are not present)

What types of equipment should be available during transfer?

- Oxygen cylinders
- Portable mechanical ventilator
- Airway equipment, e.g. endotracheal tubes and airway adjuncts
- Suction device
- IV access (ideally wide bore and bilateral ante-cubital)
- IV fluids
- Cardiac defibrillator and a back-up power source
- Drugs, e.g. to manage cardiac, respiratory, anaesthetic and full resuscitation interventions
- Monitoring equipment, e.g. continuous SaO_2, heart rate, blood pressure, respiratory rate, temperature and ECG recording

How is the patient prepared prior to transfer?

- Securing haemodynamic stability

- Securing respiratory stability, i.e. the portable ventilator should meet the needs of the patient. If there is a chest drain *in situ* its position must be checked and the underwater seal drain must be well placed
- Stabilising body temperature, e.g. controlling pyrexia and preventing hypothermia
- Requirements for sedation, muscle relaxation and analgesia must also be addressed

Procedures

Tracheostomy

Give some indications for tracheostomy
- To maintain a patent airway in congenital defects of the face or upper airway, e.g. laryngotracheomalacia, laryngeal stenosis or cysts
- To maintain a patent airway following acquired pathologies, e.g. laryngeal tumours, post-laryngectomy, diphtheria
- To maintain a patent airway in the emergency setting, e.g. laryngeal and upper airway trauma, laryngeal oedema, foreign body obstruction, inhalation injury
- To permit long-term positive pressure ventilation in those who are intubated for >2–3 weeks
- To facilitate airway suction
- To decrease the work of breathing and reduction of anatomic dead space, e.g. severe COPD, obstructive sleep apnoea

What kinds of tracheostomy do you know?
Surgical

- *Open procedure*: there is dissection in the mid-line following division and ligation of the thyroid isthmus. A vertical incision is made between the 2nd, 3rd and 4th tracheal rings. Alternatively, the trachea may have a window cut into it, or opened by lifting a flap of cartilage (Bjork flap). These two latter methods increase the risk of subsequent stenosis

Non-surgical

- *Percutaneous tracheostomy*: a small skin crease incision is placed midway between the cricoid and sternal notch. A guide wire is advanced through a 14-G cannula that has been passed through the incision. Dilators of increasing diameter are sequentially passed through to widen the aperture. Alternatively, dilating forceps widen the tracheostomy, so that the tube can be inserted into the correct position. Fibre optic bronchoscopy can be used to aid placement
- *Translaryngeal tracheostomy*: a guide wire is passed into the mouth via a cannula that pierces the trachea. The cuffed tube is passed into the mouth and fed over the wire and into the trachea, part exiting through the anterior tracheal wall
- *Minitracheostomy*: a 4 mm diameter uncuffed tube is passed through the median cricothyroid ligament under local anaesthetic. It permits regular tracheal suction and high-flow jet ventilation in the emergency setting

What problems can arise if the incision is too high or too low?
If the incision is placed too high, it can lead to subglottic stenosis; if placed too low, it can lead to a tracheoinominate fistula.

What are the advantages of a percutaneous technique?

- Can be carried out in the ICU, avoiding the operating room
- More rapid, and less traumatic, than the open method

How do tracheostomies in children differ from those in adults?

In children, low placement should be avoided due to the high risk of injury to the left brachiocephalic vein that may run above the sternal notch. Access to the tracheal lumen should be performed through a vertical slit, and removal of cartilage leads to tracheal stenosis. Cuffed tubes should generally be avoided in children because of the risk of mucosal ulceration and tracheal stenosis. Under 12 years of age, percutaneous tracheostomy should be avoided due to the risk of oesophageal injury.

What types of tracheostomy tubes are there?

A number of different types of tubes exist

- Metal or plastic
- Cuffed or uncuffed, e.g. cuffed reduces the risk of aspiration
- Fenestrated or unfenestrated, e.g. fenestration permits speech

What are the complications of tracheostomies?

Complications may be in the early or late stages

In the short term

- *Bleeding*: especially from the stump of the thyroid isthmus or anterior jugular vessels. Adrenaline-soaked swabs can be used to control minor ooze

- *Injury to surrounding structures*: e.g. oesophageal perforation, injury to recurrent laryngeal nerves, pleural reflections, brachiocephalic vein, subcutaneous emphysema
- *Displacement*: tube displacement and inadvertent extubation
- *Blockage*: this can occur due to encrusted secretions

In the medium term

- *Infection*: this ranges from superficial wound problems to severe complications, e.g. tracheitis
- *Fistula formation*: e.g. tracheoinominate fistula if erosion occurs into this local structure. This presents as a severe haemorrhage

In the long term

- *Ulceration*: mucosal ulceration and tracheal stenosis can occur if the trachoestomy is left *in situ* for prolonged periods

Once in place, how are tracheostomy tubes cared for?
Care of the tube is top priority

- *Security*: the tube must be secured in place
- *Prophylaxis*: broad spectrum antibiotics are commenced for a few days
- *Oxygen*: humidified oxygen is given for the first few days

The cuffed tube is changed to an uncuffed tube after several days, and requires regular cleaning to prevent the build-up of encrusted secretions. This involves the removal of the inner tube and cleaning in a solution such as hydrogen peroxide

(H_2O_2). NB. Emergency equipment should always be at the ready, e.g. suction devices, replacement tubes and tracheal dilators.

Bibliography

Benham-Hermetz J, Lambert M, Stephens RCM. Core training: cardiovascular failure, inotropes and vasopressors. *British Journal of Hospital Medicine.* 2012;73(5):C74–7.

Eddleston J, Goldhill D, Morris J. Levels of critical care for adult patients. Intensive Care Society Standards. London, The Intensive Care Society; 2009:1–14.

Krishna M, Zacharowski K. Principles of intra-aortic balloon pump counterpulsation. Continuing education in anaesthesia. *Critical Care and Pain Journal.* 2009;9(1):24–8.

NHS Kidney Care. *Kidney Disease: Key Facts and Figures*; 2010: 1–40.

Royal College of Surgeons of England. Renal failure, prevention and management. In *Care of the Critically Ill Surgical Patient (CCrISP®)*, 3rd edn. London, Royal College of Surgeons of England; 2010: Chapter 9.

INDEX